PATHWAYS TO NURSING

A Guide to Library and Online Research in Nursing and Allied Health

Dennis C. Tucker, Ph.D., M.A.T., M.L.S.

and

Paula Craig, M.L.S.

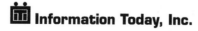 **Information Today, Inc.**

Medford, New Jersey

First printing, 2004

Pathways to Nursing: A Guide to Library and Online Research in Nursing and Allied Health

Printed and bound in the United States of America

Library of Congress Cataloging-in-Publication Data

Tucker, Dennis C.
    Pathways to nursing : a guide to library and online research in nursing and allied health /
  Dennis C. Tucker and Paula Craig.
      p. ; cm.
    Includes bibliographical references and index.
    ISBN 1-57387-192-3 (pbk.)
  1. Nursing–Research. 2. Online library catalogs. 3. Library information networks. 4. Nursing.
[DNLM: 1. Nursing Research–methods. 2. Libraries, Medical. 3. Library Services. 4. Online
Systems. WY 20.5 T891p 2004] I. Craig, Paula. II. Title.

   RT81.5.T833 2004
   610.73' 072–dc22

                              2003021856

Authors' Note:
At the risk of appearing insensitive to gender-neutral language issues, in most cases we have chosen to use masculine references as "gender-generic" rather than the cumbersome he/she, him/her, etc. When all is said and done, a book reads more smoothly written the old-fashioned way.

Publisher: Thomas H. Hogan, Sr.
Editor-in-Chief: John B. Bryans
Managing Editor: Deborah R. Poulson
Graphics Department Director: M. Heide Dengler
Copy Editor: Pat Hadley-Miller
Cover Designer: Lisa Boccadutre
Indexer: Sharon Hughes

R   SITY

Contents

Figures

Introduction

A wise person once said, "Give a man a fish and you feed him for a day; teach him to fish and you feed him for a lifetime."

Educators have often been told that we teach people, not subjects. Yet, if we teach a person a subject, we still have not fulfilled our mission. We must teach him how to learn more about that subject without assistance from us. He needs to progress beyond the limit of our knowledge. A good foundation in research skills is, therefore, an essential part of a good education and one that will last a lifetime.

Years of experience both in teaching and in library work have shown us that we educators have often failed in teaching research skills. It is the purpose of this book to provide instruction in the basic skills necessary for doing research in the area of nursing and allied health sciences. We are going to look at libraries and how they can be used to the best advantage. We will attempt to offer some basic resources and techniques that can be used by the student of nursing while in school and by the graduate—the nurse practitioner, the supervisor, the hospital worker, the clinical nurse—who no longer has access to a teacher or faculty member for direction but must gather information independently.

We will discuss, explain, and demonstrate six major components essential to the responsible development of information retrieval and utilization skills in the field of nursing and health sciences.

FIRST, we will look at the overall layout of the library itself (whether a college, university, or public library). We will discuss the organization of the holdings and their various categories and functions. We will list and explain the various staff positions typical in a library, and we will make some references to general policies of utilization commonly found in libraries.

SECOND, we will examine the library catalog, and its smaller unit, the catalog record. Each record contains a wealth of information that many nonlibrarians don't even know exists and which can serve as a springboard to a vast pool of other resources.

THIRD, we will consider the reference collection and briefly discuss what distinguishes a reference book from a nonreference book. At the same time, we will outline some basic criteria for evaluating a reference work and look at some of the major reference sources in the subject area of nursing and health sciences.

FOURTH, the professional who wishes to keep current in his field must know how to use the periodical literature to locate the latest research. We will look at periodicals and their indexes—both the traditional print indexes and their newer counterparts, electronic indexes.

FIFTH, we'll look at the Internet, the World Wide Web, and other electronic resources. We'll look at some criteria for evaluating them, examining the various types of resources, and see how they compare.

FINALLY, we will briefly discuss and illustrate an effective method of research documentation and discuss ways of developing a research paper from the choice of the initial topic to its completion.

Along the way, we will take a look at the most valuable library resource of all—the library staff, and, especially, the reference librarian. This information professional is a trained researcher with skills that will allow him or her to locate information in any field, be it theology, philosophy, medicine, law, or engineering. Nowadays, the well-prepared reference librarian is not only a researcher, but also an expert in logic (Boolean, to be precise), information management, and computer systems.

Chapter One

The Library
as a Physical Space

One of the first things the researcher will want to do is to find a library, whether it's an academic or a public library. Once you have located the library, we suggest a visit just to have a look around. Browse to get a general idea of the layout. Locate the various stack areas and the different types of collections that are contained within the building. Find the bathrooms and water fountains and the quiet areas for study. Perhaps now is a good time to locate a favorite hideaway that will later become your special secret place for studying.

Some libraries will have printed brochures that give information on the library, telling about its various collections, special display areas, where the various parts of the collection are located, etc. If such a brochure is not readily visible, ask the library personnel if one is available.

Other libraries are even more elaborate in orienting new users to the library. An increasing number of libraries are using audio or videocassettes for orientation. It is sometimes possible to check out a video for home use. Other times, the library may have a special viewing area where you can go to watch the tape, which is, in essence, a guided tour of the building and its collections. Some libraries have audiotapes that you can borrow along with a cassette player for in-house use. These tapes contain a self-guided tour of the library. You play the tape and follow its directions for a walking tour of the building.

Some libraries have personnel who will give a guided tour of the building. Depending on the policy of the library, a tour may be available at any time on request or only at scheduled times, in which case you can sign up to come back later and join a group. Most colleges and universities have some type of library tour (often called "bibliographic instruction tour").

The introductory visit to the library is a good time to get acquainted with its particular policies and procedures. What types of materials can be checked out? For how long? How do you get a library card? What types of materials must be used in-house? What are the library hours? Is there an after-hours study area? What is the availability of special collections, interlibrary loan, and computer databases? The more the researcher knows about the building and its layout, the more comfortable he will feel using its services and dealing with its personnel.

A good library contains more than just books. It will have a variety of educational materials, aids, and services with a staff of professionally trained individuals who are happy to assist the inquiring researcher seeking to utilize its resources.

There is logic to the arrangement of the materials and the organization of the various functions of the staff. The serious researcher needs to become acquainted with the library, its methods, concepts, and procedures.

At this point, it will be helpful to point out the fundamental structure of the holdings and the staff positions of the typical library. Just as not everyone who works in a doctor's office is a doctor, neither is everyone who works in a library a librarian. Just as you would not expect the doctor's receptionist to perform surgery, you should not expect a library page to have the answer to an involved research question.

Within the library are clerks, staff assistants, secretaries, pages, student workers, and librarians. The librarian is a professional with a minimum of an accredited master's degree in library science. Most institutions of higher education have the same requirements for a librarian as for a member of the teaching faculty. A second master's degree is often required for tenure.

Libraries are organized in many different ways, depending on their size and the needs of the patrons or institution they serve. But, generally speaking, libraries are organized into two broad areas: technical services and public services.

Technical Services

Technical services staff can be thought of as those who work behind the scenes. They are the people responsible for ordering the materials (though not necessarily deciding which materials to order) and handling them from the time they arrive at the delivery dock until they are on the shelf. Technical services is divided into several major areas.

Acquisitions. Those in the acquisitions department actually place the orders for the materials with the various publishers and suppliers. When the materials arrive, it is their responsibility to receive them, make sure that the order has arrived as requested, and disperse the invoices for payment and the materials for processing.

Cataloging. The cataloging department is responsible for the organization of the collection. Its duty is to see that materials on the same subject are grouped together on the shelf to make it easier for the patron to find them. Therefore, the staff classifies the materials and assigns call numbers according to whichever classification system the library uses. (In the U.S., that is usually the Dewey Decimal system, the Library of Congress system, or the National Library of Medicine system.)

The cataloging department is responsible for preparing entries for each item for the card catalog or the automated catalog and filing the cards in the drawers or adding the information to the database. Catalogers are also responsible for the process in reverse—removing entries from the catalog for materials that have been lost or discarded.

Processing. Some libraries have a processing department that is responsible for the physical preparation of the material. Processors do such tasks as applying spine labels and barcodes, inserting book pockets, and placing plastic jackets on the books.

Mending and binding. This department, sometimes combined with and sometimes separate from processing, is responsible for the physical well being of the materials. Worn and torn materials are mended and repaired. While larger libraries may have their own in-house bindery, most libraries send materials needing extensive repair to an outside bindery. It is the responsibility of this department to get them there and back.

Serials. Serials are materials that come at repeated intervals—such as yearbooks or magazines. This department is responsible for receiving the materials when they arrive, checking them in, and getting them to the shelf. It is also their responsibility to notice materials that fail to arrive and contact the supplier. In large libraries, periodicals (magazines and journals) may be a separate department from or a subdivision of the serials department.

Public Services

The people in the public services are the ones you will usually see in your visits to the library. Their primary function is to assist you, the patron.

Circulation. One of the major subdivisions of the public services department is the circulation department. This department is primarily responsible for checking out materials to the borrower and getting them back. When materials are returned, it is their job to get them back to the proper shelf. If the library uses a fine system, they must collect the fines for overdue materials. If materials are not returned, it is the responsibility of the circulation department to contact the recalcitrant borrower and, occasionally, turn over the case to a collection agency.

Reserve. The reserve book department may be contained within or be separate from the circulation department. A professor may make a reading assignment for an entire class (or several classes) in the same book. If there is only one copy of the book in the library and someone checks it out, no one else gets a chance to read the assignment. To avoid this, the professor may choose to place the book on reserve. Reserve simply means that the book is placed on limited circulation. Instead of being checked out for the usual two, three, or four weeks at a time (whatever the policy of the library is), the book may now be checked out only for overnight use or for two hours use within the library. (Again, this time period varies according to the policy of each library and the wishes of the professor.) Its purpose is to make a limited number of materials available to the greatest number of users in the shortest period of time.

Reference. The reference department is probably the department (other than circulation) that the researcher will deal with most often. Though some people find it difficult to believe, libraries actually pay someone for sitting at a desk and answering questions. This person is available and waiting to be asked.

The reference librarian is one of the most highly trained individuals in the library. He or she knows the collection and the tools for accessing it. The reference librarian with a second master's degree may also be a scholar in his own particular academic discipline. He can be the researcher's single most valuable asset.

While it is impossible for an individual reference librarian to be an expert in every single subject area in which someone may require assistance, he is trained in the techniques of locating and evaluating information. Though the sources are not the same for all disciplines, the techniques are. The reference librarian is trained in the basic sources for all disciplines or at least knows which tools to use to find them. Larger libraries have a staff of reference librarians, each with his own subject specialty; if one reference librarian can't help, possibly another one can.

Before approaching the reference librarian, there is a basic supposition that must be understood: This individual is there to help you do your work, not to do it for you.

Exhaust your own resources before asking for assistance so that you may say, "I've looked in the catalog for books on the pulmonary dysfunction, but I couldn't find any. Am I looking under the right subject heading?" rather than, "Do you have any books about the lungs?"

Expect the reference librarian to answer your question with a question. He is trained to elicit as much information from you as possible so that he may be as specific as possible in finding the answer you want. He is not trying to pry, only to be specific. If the information you are researching is confidential, say so. Reference librarians don't care what you are researching, but they do need as much information as you can give them so they can be sure of finding the right answer for you.

After the librarian has helped you, if the answer is not what you need, feel free to say, "Thank you, but that's not quite what I'm looking for. Is there another source that we could check?" The reference librarian wants to find the answer but often doesn't know if he's succeeded unless you tell him.

Be courteous in your use of the reference librarian's time. The reference desk, particularly in an academic library, can be extremely busy. It is not unusual in some libraries to see four or five people in line and two phones ringing at the same time. Try to keep your query as brief and simple as possible. If your question requires an in-depth answer that is going to take some time, schedule your time at the reference desk when it is less busy. Some reference desks will even make an appointment for you to have a lengthy session with the person who is most skilled in your subject area.

Undergraduate students are known for not beginning their work on time. Reference librarians hear a favorite complaint of teachers even more often: "I have this term paper due tomorrow and I need five sources." Locating information takes time. After it is found, it most likely will not be in the form needed for the final paper or project. It is going to take some time for the researcher to pull it together and reorganize it. The responsibility of the reference librarian ends with locating the information; pulling it all together in final form is the responsibility of the student or researcher.

It is fair to expect the reference librarian to teach you how to use the catalog or to show you where the materials are found. It is not fair to ask the librarian to look up every book or to retrieve it for you. If you don't understand something about the library, ask, but ask with the goal of learning to do it for yourself.

Telephone reference. Many libraries offer telephone reference service. These libraries will take a phone call and give you a specific piece of information over the phone. By all means, use the service, but do not abuse it.

Keep your phone query to a simple fact or two. The telephone reference staff will be glad to tell you the current population of Paris or whether or not the library has a certain book (and in some cases whether it is checked out or not), but do not expect them to have time to read you a four-page essay over the phone.

If it sounds like the library is busy, keep your phone query brief or ask if there is a more convenient time for you to call back. Traffic at the reference desk goes in spurts: The librarian may sit for 10 or 15 minutes with no questions and suddenly six people approach at the same time—all of them with lengthy requests. Most libraries give priority to the patron who has put forth the effort to go in person over the one making a convenient phone call from home. For questions that are lengthy, some libraries will be glad to take your phone number and call you back.

Interlibrary loan. If the library doesn't own the book you need or seems to have nothing on your topic, ask the reference librarian if they have interlibrary loan service. This service provides access to books from other libraries where you would not normally be allowed borrowing privileges. Again, be as specific as possible with your request. Some libraries will only handle a request for a specific book, while others are prepared to fill a more general request for "any information" on a given topic.

Always allow two to three weeks for an interlibrary loan request. Remember that your library is at the mercy of the lending library, so do not get upset with your library if the book is slow in coming. Ask what the usual response time is; then, if you haven't heard by that time, inquire again.

If the length of time you may keep the material is short, that time has been determined by the lending library, not by your library. If renewals are not allowed, that is the policy of the lender, not of your library.

Online reference. Another department under the umbrella of public services may be the online reference department. It may be called "Online Searching," "Information Retrieval," or a myriad of other names. Many of the indexes, which were previously available only in paper form, plus many new ones, are now available in electronic format. Depending on the complexity of your search and the type of information you need, this may be the quickest and best way to locate the information. If you think you might need the service, ask if it's available. For more information on online searching, see the section "Online Search Services" in Chapter 5.

Bibliographic instruction. Larger libraries often have a department devoted specifically to bibliographic instruction—teaching about books and libraries, your library in particular. It is this department that conducts the orientation tours for the new students and provides materials to professors for use in teaching about the library in the classroom. If you want to learn how to use the library to your best advantage, someone from this department can work with you.

Periodicals. Another major department is periodicals. We discussed previously the subdivision of the periodicals department that is responsible for receiving the materials and getting them to the shelves. This is the subdivision which handles the materials once they are on the shelf and available to the user.

Periodicals are generally divided into two sections: current periodicals and bound periodicals (older issues).

Current periodicals. In many libraries, the current issues are in an area by themselves. Many libraries simply place the materials on the shelf in alphabetical order by the title of the magazine or journal. Some libraries, however, classify them and assign a call number so that all journals on the same subject are shelved near each other. In this case, you will need to use a catalog to find the call number so you can locate the journal.

The type of catalog used for journals varies from library to library. Some libraries simply keep a printed list or a computer printout listing the journals that are held. Often, additional information is given, such as the volume numbers and dates of each title owned by the library. Other libraries use a "visible file," which is a kind of chart listing the titles in alphabetical sequence. Each title is held in a strip of plastic and the chart may be updated with relative ease as titles are added or dropped. Still other libraries list their journals in the main library catalog so that the user may go there to find out if the library owns a particular title.

Bound periodicals. Older materials are often moved to a separate area of the library.[1] Some libraries bind their magazines so that the issues stay together and are easier to shelve and locate. To many new users the shelves look like they are full of books, but a glance inside the covers will show that they are just the magazines we are familiar with, sewn together at the spine, and with a hard, booklike cover added to them.

Other libraries simply box the materials so that the issues of a given volume are shelved together in the same box. Some libraries discard their paper copies of journals altogether and keep back issues only on microfilm or microfiche.

Within a given library, it is not unusual to find materials treated all four ways: some bound, some boxed, some on microfilm, and some on microfiche.

Depending on the library, the section for bound journals may be a special section housing only journals, as is often the case. Some libraries, however, classify and catalog the older issues just as they would a book. So, a nursing journal will be found shelved in the regular stacks right next to the nursing books.

Periodicals indexes. Somewhere near the periodicals you will usually find the periodicals indexes. If you are trying to find an article on pressure sores, for example, you could just go to a journal where you think the article might have appeared and flip through issues until you found it, but such a procedure would probably require a great deal of time and effort unless you were sure of the exact journal and knew the issue in which it appeared. A much easier way is to locate a periodicals index and look under "pressure sores" or whatever subject you need to locate. There, you will find the title of the journal the article appeared in, its author, the issue it appeared in, and the numbers of the pages on which it appeared. We will discuss periodicals indexes in greater depth in Chapter 4.

Government documents. Many libraries, especially larger ones, have a collection of government documents. Despite the awe-inspiring title, these are nothing more than a collection of items that are published by federal, state, and local government entities. Each year government organizations publish thousands of documents. Some libraries are defined as "depository libraries," which means they automatically receive all or a selected portion of these items. Because there are so many items, it could be a time-consuming and overwhelming task to classify all of them and add them to the regular collection. So, some libraries simply designate a special area for them and use the classification scheme that has been established by the government. While quite different from the Dewey or Library of Congress systems, it is no more difficult, and the researcher should learn to use it early on if he will need government publications in the research process—and chances are most of us will.

In addition to the previously mentioned departments, which are in most every library, your library may have other special departments. Sometimes these are classed under the title of Special Collections and may include rare books, the university archives, denominational archives (if the institution is affiliated with a particular religious body), the collected works of a particular author, a genealogy collection, or a local history collection. There are many types of special collections, and some may be unique to an institution. Ask which ones your library has.

Endnote

1. The definition of "older" varies widely from one library to another, but, very generally, it means anything prior to the current year.

Chapter Two

The Library Catalog

Just as the telescope allows us to pick out and focus on a particular star in the heavens, so the library catalog is an instrument that allows us to pick out and focus on the information we need from within the vast resources of the library.

The library catalog provides multiple points of access to the library collection: The primary points are author, title, and subject. Some libraries have an online catalog that also allows searching by keyword. Let us look first at the traditional card catalog.

The Card Catalog

Some libraries use a dictionary-style card catalog in which all three types of cards—author, title, and subject—are filed in a single alphabet. Other libraries use a divided catalog with each type of card filed in a separate alphabet in a separate cabinet or set of cabinets. In other libraries, author and title cards are filed together and subject cards are filed in a separate alphabet. It is vital for the researcher to know which type of system a library uses before beginning research.

It is also important to know which style of filing system the library uses. Most libraries use word-by-word filing and follow a rule called the "nothing before something" rule. In a word-by-word system, for example, the subject "New York" would file before "Newark" or "Newsweek" because nothing—the blank space between the two words—files before something—the letter "a" or the letter "s." This rule is becoming increasingly important to understand with the advent of automation because a computer will alphabetize "nothing" before "something."

Another important filing rule is the "by before about" rule. All the books by an author are filed in the catalog before books about him. Likewise, a book written by "Brown, Zelda" would file before a book entitled *The Brown Boat.*

There is also a hierarchy of filing rules as to which comes first of commas, periods, colons, semicolons, and hyphens. Generally, a library user need not be concerned with such intricate detail other than to know that if you do not find the book listed where you think it should be, try another likely spot. If you have trouble locating a book, inquire which system your library uses or ask the reference librarian for help.

The Catalog Card

The individual unit of the catalog is the catalog card. Being able to read and understand the information contained on a card will unleash great research power.

A card is divided into paragraphs, as shown in Figure 2.1. Each paragraph is indented and contains specific information. Author, title, and subject cards are virtually alike, but different information is printed at the top of the card.

Author. Figure 2.1 is a sample of a catalog card for *Transcultural Nursing: Assessment and Intervention.* The first paragraph of a catalog card always begins with the last name of the author (1), if there is an author. This card is what we call an author card. Note that the birth and death dates of the author are sometimes given (2). This helps the researcher distinguish between people of the same name. (Try looking in the catalog of a large library for John Kennedy.) The author card is usually called the

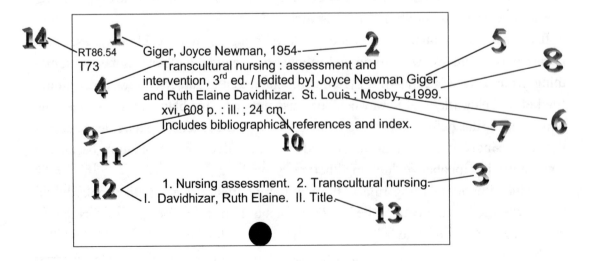

Figure 2.1   Catalog card for *Transcultural Nursing*

"main entry" and may sometimes contain more information than a similar title or subject card. When there is no author, the title of the work appears first and the title card is considered the main entry.

Subject. If this were a subject card, the subject "Nursing assessment" (3) would be written at the very top of the card above the author paragraph in all capital letters. Some catalogs still contain older cards on which the subjects were typed at the top using red ink, but current practice is to use all caps. Either red ink or all-caps indicates that this is the subject, not the title, of the book. A subject may be a topic per se, or it may be the name of a person, place, or thing.

Title. Below the author's name, and indented, is the title of the book (4). If this were a title card, the title would be repeated at the top of the card above the author's name. Note that the title is neither typed in red nor in all capital letters and that only the first word and proper nouns are capitalized. (This style of noncapitalization is followed simply to increase the cataloger's typing speed by not having to press the "shift" key repeatedly.)

Statement of Responsibility. Immediately following the title and in the same paragraph is what is called the statement of responsibility, which is usually a repetition of the author's name and may include co-authors (5), editors, or illustrators. Next, and in the same paragraph, is the imprint. The imprint is information specific to this edition of the book. If this is at least the second edition of a book, it will list here which edition this is. The imprint contains the publisher's name (6) and location (7) and the copyright date of the book (8). The researcher can use information from the imprint to determine the nationality of a publication. A book published in Ireland may not give a proper perspective of some American event, but it may be the best source for something that occurred in Ireland. A glance at the publisher's name may tell the researcher something about the quality of this book, and the copyright date will show how current the information is.

Collation. The paragraph after the imprint is the collation. If the paragraph begins with a lowercase Roman numeral, that tells how many pages of introductory material are contained in the work. An Arabic numeral (9) shows the number of pages in the body of the work. The statement "il.," "ill.," or "illus." indicates that the book contains illustrations. If you must have a picture of the person or subject you are researching and this statement is absent, obviously you should look for another source. Often the statement is so specific as to indicate that the book contains maps, charts, graphs, or other specific types of illustrative material. Finally, many cards give the height of the book in centimeters (10). Generally of interest to librarians for shelving purposes, this statement may give you an overall idea of the size of the book. You won't want to plan on walking home or riding the bus with a stack of books that are 96 centimeters tall.

Notes. Following the collation is the notes paragraph (11). If the book has an index or a bibliography, it is listed here. Many cards list the page number on which this information is given. With this information, a researcher can quickly locate a book, which he might have bypassed as being of no value for his project, but the bibliography may prove invaluable in locating further sources (or "primary" or original sources) on the subject. Some cards may give additional notes about the work, such as a brief summary of the book or some type of information particular to this edition, or even information such as "autographed by the author." This note on *Transcultural Nursing* shows that it includes bibliographical references and an index.

Tracings. The last paragraph on the card is called the tracing (12). Those items that appear following Arabic numerals are subject headings under which this book is listed in the card catalog (3). They are extremely helpful to the researcher wishing to locate similar books or other books on the same topic. Simply make note of what seems to be a promising subject heading and look in the catalog under that heading. Items that appear after Roman numerals (13) are called "added entries" and refer to such things as co-authors, illustrators, alternate titles, or the series of which the book forms a part, if any. The researcher who wants to find similar books might want to look elsewhere in the catalog under the name of the co-author or the series.

Call number. Finally, in the upper left-hand corner of the card is the "call number" (14), which tells where the book is located on the shelf. In most libraries in the U.S., this number will belong either to the Dewey Decimal system, the Library of Congress system, or the National Library of Medicine (NLM) classification system, based on the *W* schedule, which the Library of Congress reserves for NLM use.

A Dewey number will have a first line that consists of numerals only with exactly three digits to the left of the decimal point. The second line is a Cutter number, which is a mixture of letters and numbers representing the author's last name and the title of the work. Generally speaking, a Cutter number will begin with a capital letter (the first letter of the author's last name) followed by two or three digits, followed by a lower case letter, which is the first letter of the first significant word of the title. Some libraries simply use the first three letters of the author's last name instead of a true Cutter number. Sometimes the Cutter number may be based on the title of the work.

A typical Dewey call number would appear like this:

Subject number	618.2
Cutter number	M484r

A Library of Congress (LC) number or an NLM number will consist of a subject number, comprising letters and numerals and a Cutter number. An LC or NLM number always begins with a letter or two. The Cutter number is preceded by a decimal point. (An LC number may contain several decimal points, while a Dewey number may contain only one.) A typical LC would appear thus:

Subject number	PS 613
Cutter number	.W47

A typical NLM would appear thus (with an LC number first):

Subject number	WY49
Cutter number	.C294h

In both systems the Cutter number is treated as a decimal, so on the shelf a book with the LC number "PS613.W47" would come before "PS613.W5." A book with the Dewey number "618.2 M484r" would come before "618.2 M53j."

For an introduction to the library and classification systems, the researcher is well advised to take a careful look at Jean Key Gates's *Guide to the Use of Libraries and Information Sources,* 7th edition (New York: McGraw-Hill, 1994) and the *Dewey Decimal Classification and Relative Index,* Edition 22 (Dublin, OH: Online Computer Library Center, 2003).

The Library of Congress Classification System

The task of recataloging and reclassifying the Library of Congress began in 1897. The Library of Congress Classification System, which was developed in that process, combines letters of the alphabet and Arabic numerals; it provides for the most minute groupings of subjects through the combination of letters and numerals; it is designed for libraries with very large collections. The letters I, O, W, X, and Y are not used but are left for further expansion or are used in complementary classification systems such as the National Library of Medicine.

A brief outline of the Library of Congress Classification System follows:

A   General Works
B   Philosophy, Psychology, Religion
C   Auxiliary Sciences of History
D   History: General and Old World
E–F History: America
G   Geography, Anthropology, Recreation
H   Social Sciences
J   Political Science
K   Law
L   Education
M   Music and Books on Music
N   Fine Arts
P   Language and Literature
Q   Science
R   Medicine
S   Agriculture
T   Technology
U   Military Science
V   Naval Science
Z   Library Science

The major subdivisions for nursing and health sciences are:

Subclass R	Medicine (General)
Subclass RA	Public Aspects of Medicine
Subclass RB	Pathology
Subclass RC	Internal Medicine
Subclass RD	Surgery
Subclass RE	Ophthalmology
Subclass RF	Otorhinolaryngology
Subclass RG	Gynecology and Obstetrics
Subclass RJ	Pediatrics
Subclass RK	Dentistry
Subclass RL	Dermatology
Subclass RM	Therapeutics. Pharmacology
Subclass RS	Pharmacy and Materia Medica

Subclass RT	Nursing
Subclass RV	Botanic, Thomsonian, and Eclectic Medicine
Subclass RX	Homeopathy
Subclass RZ	Other Systems of Medicine

While there are many other subcategories within these divisions, these subcategories will give the researcher some exposure to the sophistication and detailed specialization that library science has brought to the cataloging of books in modern times.

The Dewey Decimal Classification System

In the Dewey Decimal classification system, Arabic numerals are used to signify the various classes of subjects. It was created by an early American librarian, Melvil Dewey, who divided all knowledge, as represented by books and other materials, into nine classes, which he numbered 100 to 900. Materials too general to belong in a specific group, such as encyclopedias, dictionaries, newspapers, handbooks, and the like, he placed in a 10th class, which precedes the others as the 000 class. Every researcher should know these 10 categories. They are part of the basic knowledge of research, and the researcher will use this information at every library using the Dewey Decimal classification system. These 10 major categories are:

000	General Works
100	Philosophy
200	Religion
300	Social Sciences
400	Language
500	Pure Science
600	Technology, Applied Science
700	The Arts
800	Literature
900	History, Biography

The system progresses from the preceding 10 general classifications to increasingly precise subclassifications, based on a decade arrangement. Each of the previously mentioned 10 categories is again divided into 10 subcategories, thus providing 100 slots into which books may be classified. Each of these 100 slots is again divided into 10 further classification areas.

Usually, this three-digit *thousand* category is followed by a decimal point, after which the subdividing continues. Materials of interest for nursing can be found in the larger categories of Humanities, Medicine, or other areas.

Both systems are simply ways of classifying information so that books on a given topic are placed near each other on the shelf. This, in turn, makes it easier for the user to locate other books on the chosen subject. While smaller libraries tend to use Dewey and larger libraries LC, there is no rule, and it actually makes little difference to the user.

Some libraries handle biography and autobiography a little differently from other types of nonfiction. Instead of being assigned a call number, biographies may simply be marked with a "B" and shelved in a separate section. Other libraries use "921" or simply a "92" (from the *Dewey Decimal* system) to indicate biography. Usually biographies are filed by last name of the subject (not the author) so all biographies about Lincoln would appear together on the shelf. If biographies aren't where it seems they should be, ask where they are shelved.

Some libraries shelve fiction in a separate section. Instead of a call number, an "F" or "Fic" is given for the call number, and the books are then filed by author's last name in the fiction section. Other libraries don't bother to indicate "F" or "Fic" and the call number appears blank, indicating simply that books are filed in the fiction section by author's last name. In some libraries, some works of fiction may be classified as literature and shelved with the regular collection under the appropriate call number for literature.

Where do you begin if you don't know what the proper subject heading is for a topic? How do you know whether to look under "Railroad trains," "Trains," "Trains, Railroad," "Passenger trains," "Passenger service—rail," "Trains, Passenger," or "Railroads, Passenger"? If library catalogers filed a card under whatever subject heading appealed to them at the moment, it would be difficult to locate all the books in the library on a given subject, particularly if there were staff changes in the cataloging department over the years. Therefore, catalogers use a guide entitled *Library of Congress Subject Headings* (*LCSH*) for the express purpose of providing standardization. If you're not sure what the proper subject heading is, look in *LCSH*—a large red book, usually in two volumes—under what you feel is the most likely subject heading. *LCSH* provides ample cross-references to the correct heading. (Proper headings are printed in **Boldface** print.) Many libraries keep a copy of *LCSH* near the library catalog or at the reference desk. If you do not see a copy of *LCSH*, ask at the reference desk.

The Online Catalog

Many libraries have now automated their catalogs. Automation allows greater flexibility in manipulating information and a larger number of access points for the user. Some systems even contain circulation information so the user knows immediately if the desired book is on the shelf or checked out. Often the information on the computer screen will look similar to that on a catalog card. All the information available on a catalog card is available on the screen of an online system (see Figures 2.2 and 2.3). There is no standardized format for online data, so the researcher must learn to locate the desired information on whatever system is in use.

The online catalog has several advantages over the card catalog. First of all, the online catalog is easier to maintain. While that would seem to be of no consequence to the researcher, it is an important advantage. Because keeping a card catalog updated (inserting new cards and removing those for lost or discarded items) is very labor-intensive, the card catalog is seldom truly updated. The online catalog, however, may

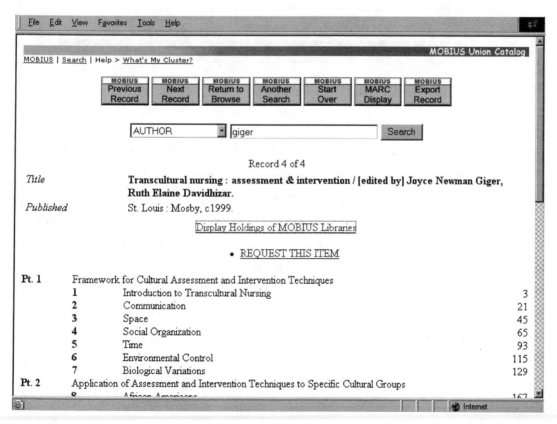

Figure 2.2   OPAC entry for *Transcultural Nursing*

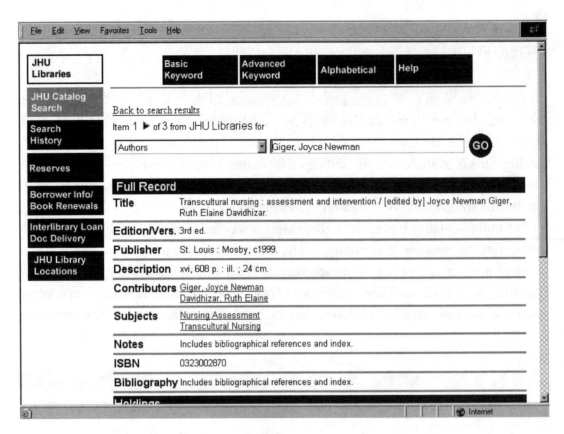

Figure 2.3   OPAC entry for *Transcultural Nursing*

be up-to-the-minute because the cataloging librarian can create the electronic record for an item and instantly add it to the database. Likewise, missing or discarded items can be promptly removed from the database.

The online catalog harnesses the power of the computer for the researcher's advantage. In the traditional card catalog, the researcher had only three entry points: the name of the author, the title of the work, or the subject of the work. A researcher trying to locate a specific work in a card catalog must know either its author or its title. Furthermore, he must know the first word of the title. In order to locate the *Handbook of Nursing Diagnosis* in the card catalog, the researcher would have to know that the first word of the title is "Handbook." Looking under "Nursing" or "Diagnosis" would yield many results as subject headings, but not necessarily the title he is seeking. In the online catalog, however, the researcher could enter any of those words or some combination and likely locate the work quickly and easily.

An online catalog allows many other entry points; for example, keywords from a particular part of the record (called a *field*) or from all fields. As in the title search mentioned previously, if the researcher has some idea what the work is about he can search for keywords from the subject field. For example, to locate the *Handbook of Nursing Diagnosis* in the online catalog, the researcher could search for the keywords "nursing" and "diagnosis" in the subject field without having to know that the exact "approved" subject heading is "Nursing Diagnosis—Handbooks."

The online catalog allows the researcher to limit the search. For example, if the researcher knows that the word "dictionary" appears in the title of the work, he could limit the search for the word specifically to the title field, thereby excluding all those works that had the word "dictionary" only in the subject field.

The online catalog allows the user to search many fields that could not be indexed in the traditional card catalog, for example the "notes" field. This field often contains a short summary or abstract of the work and may contain important clues to locating it. By searching the notes, the researcher may be able to locate a book that he would not have been able to find in a card catalog.

Fields can be combined in specific ways in an online search. For example, the search can specify that the work must contain the name "Melton" in the author field and the word "American" in the title field.

Searches may also be limited in order to find more easily works germane to the topic. A search can be limited by date (e.g., works prior to 1956) or by language (e.g., works in German only). Some catalogs allow searching or limiting by other fields such as publisher, place of publication, or even the number of pages.

In brief, the online catalog allows the user to tailor a search to locate only those resources most relevant to the research topic.

Another item of information given in the online catalog is shelf status of the sought-after work. The researcher can tell while still at the catalog if the work is on the shelf, checked out (and, sometimes, when it is due back), missing, or on order. The user of the card catalog, meanwhile, must note the location of each item and go to the library shelves to see if it is available. If the item is not on the shelf, he must then ask the library staff if the item is checked out, missing, etc. The online catalog will save the researcher much time and frustration.

If the needed item is not on the shelf, the researcher using an online catalog can often place a hold on the item. Thus, when it is returned to the library, the library staff will notify the researcher that the item is now available. Some automation systems will allow the user to place the hold directly; in other systems, the user must request the library staff to do it on his behalf.

Whichever system your library uses, introduce yourself early and become familiar with it. A couple of hours "playing" in the library will be an invaluable timesaver when there is a research deadline to be met.

Chapter Three

The Reference Collection— Tomes of Information

Due to a lack of basic research skills, a beginning researcher may assume the library deficient in materials when, in reality, there is a mountain of literature that is inaccessible to the untrained user. Nowhere in the library is there to be found such a concentration of research materials as in the reference department. Many kinds of dictionaries, encyclopedias, government documents, and a full range of indices will be found here. We will discuss these groupings later, but first, let us take a closer look at reference books in general.

Evaluating a Reference Book

What is a reference book? What distinguishes it from a nonreference book?

A primary distinction is revealed by the term itself: A reference book is not intended to be read from cover to cover like a novel or a biography, but is referred to in order to locate specific factual information. The information is usually, but not always, brief in nature.

Having determined what a reference book is, how do you determine what a *good* reference book is? There are a number of criteria that may be applied.

First of all, read the introductory material. Usually there is a section (or sections) at the beginning of the work that tells its purpose and scope and briefly outlines its contents. Knowing the authors' purpose, we can then apply other criteria to decide whether or not they fulfill that purpose.

Scope. The scope of a book is its span of coverage. To locate information efficiently we must determine whether a particular book deals adequately with the topic we are investigating. A book entitled *America in the Twenties* would probably be limited to a discussion of things happening in America during the 1920s and would not be our primary text for research on European current events during World War II. Its scope includes neither the topic we are researching (Europe) nor the time period (World War II).

Bias. Merriam-Webster defines bias as "an inclination of temperament or outlook; especially: a personal and *sometimes* unreasoned judgment."[1] Bias is not always a negative term. Bias is simply the author's feelings toward his subject. However, when an author's point of view is limited by the purposeful exclusion of any evidence that disagrees with his opinion, we can say that he is unfairly biased.

The distinction between a biased work and an unbiased one is sometimes thin, but essentially, if an author presents his viewpoint as one of several viewpoints to be considered, we can say the work is unbiased. If he presents his viewpoint as the only and absolute truth, willfully excluding or ignoring abundant evidence to the contrary, we can say the work is biased. In researching the history of a particular denomination, for example, a text written by a member of that denomination may be the best source, for a member can have a feeling and an appreciation for the denomination that an outsider cannot. If, however, the author's zeal for promoting the denomination distorts the facts, a text written by an outside party may be the best source.

Point of view. Every book has a point of view. To determine whether a book suits our research purpose, we must determine what that point of view is. The author might be looking at his subject from either the inside or the outside—a member of a denomination or an outsider writing its history. His purpose might be to convert or simply to lay down the facts. An author's timeframe is also a point of view. A book like the previously mentioned *America in the Twenties* could either be a look at current events or a historical perspective of the decade, depending on when it was written and the point of view of the author. Either point of view is valid, but one or the other may not suit our purpose. In choosing a reference book, we must make sure that the author's point of view is appropriate to the subject and to our needs.

Copyright. The copyright date of a work can often tell us immediately if it is the source we need. If the piece of information we need is the current membership of Pentecostal churches in Latin America, a book with a 1967 copyright date will give us the wrong information. Although perfectly correct when the book was published, time has made the information false if we need a current figure. On the other hand, if we are charting growth over the years, the 1967 figure may be exactly the one we need.

Index. Is the work indexed? Check the back of the book (or, rarely, the front) to see if there is an index. Many otherwise potentially useful books are worth less than the paper they are written on because the information they contain is virtually inaccessible.

Organization. Is the book organized chronologically? Geographically? Alphabetically? By topic? Poor organization can waste much of a researcher's time. If we need information on the growth of the church in Latin America, a chronological (but not geographical) organization could waste hours of our time, as we have to search through data on all the other countries of the world seeking those items that refer only to Latin America. Likewise, a strictly geographical organization might not show us the progress of growth over time. If we want to chart growth country by country, a work that gives statistics only by region will not give us the information we need. In any of these cases, it might be better to find another work whose organization more exactly fits our needs.

Author's credentials. Finally, take a look at the credentials of the author. Has he written on this topic before? What has his experience in the field been? Has he based his work on that of others who have been prominent in the field? If so, has he agreed or disagreed with them? Has he added to their discoveries, or merely rehashed them? How have others in the field regarded his work? What do the critics say? If you know that the author is someone whose viewpoint is vastly different from yours, you probably will not find much support in his works for the argument you are trying to present.

While it may require a little extra effort, taking some additional time to find the appropriate source can often represent time-savings over taking the first source that comes along.

Dictionaries

The major "unabridged" English-language dictionaries most useful to the researcher are *Webster's New International Dictionary of the English Language*, *Webster's Third New International Dictionary, Merriam-Webster OnLine* (http://www. merriamwebster.com), or *Funk and Wagnall's New Standard Dictionary*. For studying word origins, the standard is the *Oxford English Dictionary* (*OED*).

It should be noted here that "Webster's" is a generic term coming from Noah Webster, compiler of an early dictionary, and can be used by anyone. Merriam-Webster is a reputable dictionary publisher, producer of the *Third New International Dictionary* mentioned previously. If you find it confusing to distinguish one "Webster's" from another, that's just what some not-so-reputable publishers want. Just because it's a "Webster's" dictionary is no sign that it's necessarily a good one.

Major components of language dictionaries include spelling, etymologies (the history of a word), definitions, pronunciation, synonyms, syllabication, and grammatical information.

Specialized Dictionaries in Nursing and Health Sciences

In addition to language dictionaries, there is a wide range of specialized subject dictionaries that the informed researcher will want to become acquainted with, and these may be found in the reference section.

- *Dorland's Illustrated Medical Dictionary*. Philadelphia: W. B. Saunders, 1900–.
- *Miller-Keane Encyclopedia and Dictionary of Medicine, Nursing, and Allied Health*, 7th ed. Philadelphia: W. B. Saunders, 2003.
- *Taber's Cyclopedic Medical Dictionary*. Philadelphia: F. A. Davis, 1940–.
- *Mosby's Medical, Nursing, and Allied Health Dictionary*, 6th ed. St. Louis: C. V. Mosby, 2002.

Encyclopedias

There is more than one kind of encyclopedia, even though many undergraduate students have been nurtured with the notion that either the *Encyclopedia Americana* or the *World Book,* or, if the student is particularly interested in specialized knowledge, the *Encyclopaedia Britannica*, constitute the full range. Though these are very valuable sources of general information, the nursing student serious about library research will seek out specialized encyclopedias, which will prove to be the most valuable of all. Nevertheless, general encyclopedias do have a great deal of merit.

General Encyclopedias

"For your research paper, you must use three different sources and you can't use an encyclopedia." Surely, every student has heard this from his teacher numerous times during elementary and high school. Why the bias against encyclopedias? Are they inherently evil? What's wrong with them?

Actually, nothing is basically wrong with using encyclopedias—the good ones anyway—if they are used properly. But fifth graders (and sometimes university students) tend to rely on them too completely. Encyclopedias are often like distilled water—the essence is there, but not the flavor. Students use them heavily because they want their research predigested for them rather than doing it themselves from primary sources.

So, why do encyclopedias exist? Who should use them and when? How should they be used?

Encyclopedias are a ready-reference source—a handy place for quick information. They provide a broad overview of popular subjects of general interest (hence the term "general interest encyclopedia"). The articles in an encyclopedia are written by experts in the field and are aimed at those who are not.

Encyclopedias can serve the specialist by providing a summary of his or her discipline, or the novice by providing an introduction. They are a good starting point. The novice doing research on Louis XIV can get an idea of when and where he lived and who he was from the general encyclopedia. That information, at least, will tell us that we probably won't find much about him in a book on avant-garde theater in Buenos Aires, but surely will find him in books on the history of France.

If we learn from the encyclopedia that John Doe is an author and is currently living, we know to look next in reference works on contemporary authors. From the encyclopedia we learn that the Haversian canals are an anatomical, not a geographical, feature and that Menno Simons is a name we'll want to be on the lookout for while studying the history of the Mennonites.

The encyclopedia can also be useful as a bibliographic tool. Some encyclopedias list books and articles for further reading on the topic. Check the introductory material for the encyclopedia to see if bibliographies are given and if they are with the articles or in a separate section. Rather than wonder if the library has "any books on XYZ," the prepared researcher will have a list of books and can go directly to the catalog to see if the library has them.

When using the encyclopedia, always approach the topic through the index, rather than by the grammar school method of grabbing the appropriate volume and looking directly for the article. Louis XIV may be listed in the "L" volume; or he may not be. But the researcher who looks only in the "L" volume rather than in the index will surely miss many other references to him in articles on the history of France and other topics.

Use the encyclopedia. Use it often. But use it well, and use it only as a starting point for further research.

Specialized Encyclopedias in Nursing and Health Sciences

- *The Merck Manual of Diagnosis and Therapy.* Rahway, NJ: Merck, 1899–.
- Miller, Benjamin Fran and Claire B. Keane. *Encyclopedia and Dictionary of Medicine, Nursing, and Allied Health,* 7th ed. Philadelphia: W. B. Saunders, 2003.
- Schroeder, Patricia. *Encyclopedia of Nursing Care Quality.* Boston: Jones & Bartlett, 1995.
- *Encyclopedia of Nursing Research.* Joyce J. Fitzpatrick, ed. New York: Springer, 1998.
- Mezey, Mathy Doval. *The Encyclopedia of Elder Care: The comprehensive resource on geriatric and social care.* New York: Springer, 2001.
- *The Gale Encyclopedia of Nursing and Allied Health.* Detroit: Gale Group, 2002.
- *Nurse's Book of Advice: An Encyclopedia of Answers to Hundreds of Difficult Questions—Ethical, Legal, Moral, Technical, and Professional.* Springhouse, PA: Springhouse, 1992.

Government Documents

Although the government documents section of the reference collection is problematical and complex, the researcher in nursing may often need to refer to these documents. Initially, you might wish to consult one of these two sources for a general overview of the available materials: Joe Morehead's *Introduction to United States Public Documents,* 3rd ed. (Littleton, CO: Libraries Unlimited, Inc., 1983, 309 pp.) or

Laurence F. Schmeckebier and Roy B. Eastin's *Government Publications and Their Use,* 2nd revised ed., (Washington, DC: The Brookings Institute, 1986, 502 pp.).

An important tool used in locating U.S. government documents is the *Monthly Catalog of U.S. Government Publications* (U.S. Superintendent of Documents, 1895 to date) because it is the single most comprehensive listing of all unclassified publications issued by the various departments and agencies of the U.S. government. Another reference of major importance because it offers a comprehensive annotated guide to the series and periodicals produced by agencies and departments of the U.S. government is J. L. Andriot et al.'s *Guide to U.S. Government Publications* (Farmington Hills, MI, Gale Group 1973–). For further listings, library staff will be happy to show you many of these sources and their primary method of use.

Indexes

Indexes are an indispensable category of reference works for the researcher of nursing and health sciences. As these sources generally index primarily periodicals and journals—although sometimes including books and other types of material—and are often shelved with or near the periodicals, they are discussed in Chapter 4.

Endnote

1. Merriam-Webster's Collegiate Dictionary, accessed October 26, 2003: http://www.m-w.com

Chapter Four

Periodicals and Indexes

Periodicals

Some students are of the false impression that the library subscribes to magazines and newspapers just for recreational reading, that is, the magazines and various other loose items lying near and shelved close to comfortable reading desks and lounge chairs are there for the general amusement of the bored student. But that's not the total picture.

From a research and scholarly point of view, there is no such thing as serious research or scholarship in the absence of the periodical literature. Furthermore, there is a profoundly important difference between the various kinds of periodical materials subscribed to by the library. To call a scholarly journal a "magazine" is a great disservice. The scholarly journal consists of heavily researched articles of a specialized nature and published for the professionals in that field.

Magazines, on the other hand, are written for the general public, the casual reader, and are not research scholarship. Good magazine articles may be helpful in orienting the layperson and the beginning researcher to the general range and nature of a topic but would never constitute the literature foundation for a serious research project. Any serious researcher would never refer to research scholarship in the journals as "magazine" articles. Language and terminology, as always, reflect the depth of the researcher's training and awareness.

The library does more than just provide copies of the latest issues of scholarly journals. It also collects the back issues and gathers them into a special collection often held in some large chamber of the library. The periodicals, therefore, are naturally divided into two categories, often called the Current Periodicals Section or room and the Bound Periodicals Section or room.

Current periodicals. This section of the library is easily identified, for here the journals, magazines, and periodical materials to which the library subscribes may be displayed on easy-to-get-at shelves or racks arranged so that the general reader can peruse the collection, often without having to handle each item, by reading the covers of the journals where the contents may be listed in a convenient quick-to-use manner.

The current periodicals constitute the latest issues of a journal to which the library subscribes. The informed researcher will make it a frequent practice to scan all of the periodicals subscribed to by the library in her own field of study and interest. By merely reading the table of contents (often printed on the cover) of the major periodicals in the field, the researcher can keep up with the general development of ideas and activities of special personal interest.

As the current issue of a periodical is replaced by a later one, the older issue is usually placed somewhere near the latest one. Many shelves are arranged so that the older issues are kept immediately behind or under the current one. The researcher can locate them simply by lifting the shelf. These issues are kept together until a volume is accumulated and then sent off for binding and relocation in the Bound Periodicals Section. (A volume may constitute a year's worth of journals or perhaps only two or three months' worth. The most important criterion that libraries use is keeping the bound volume of manageable size.)

Bound periodicals section. There usually isn't room for the library to keep every issue of every journal to which it subscribes all together in the Current Periodicals Section, especially when one considers that there are often several hundred subscriptions and an accumulation of many decades. Therefore, it becomes necessary for the library to store the back issues of the major periodicals of the collection for easy access.

Virtually every library keeps some kind of list of its periodicals holdings. This list (which may take the form of a printed or computerized list, a card or book catalog, or a visible file) is an alphabetical listing of all the periodicals owned by the library and, just as importantly, the date the subscription commenced (and ended, if the journal is no longer received). Some collections could go back a hundred years, while others will date much more recently. This information is crucial, for it tells the researcher immediately whether or not a particular periodical is available in the library and at what point the subscription began (and ended).

In addition, the holdings list will describe in what form the back issues are kept. There is no use looking on the shelves if the issues are kept only in microform. Microform may be microfilm or microfiche. Some libraries may use film, while others will use fiche, and some use both. It is extremely important that the researcher know in which form the issues are kept, for that information will determine where they are located. Though sometimes located on the shelves with the bound materials, microfilm and microfiche are usually filed in special cabinets and may be kept in a special area of the library. Because of differences in shape and size, film and fiche are usually kept in separate cabinets.

Let us illustrate the importance of this listing. Say a researcher has found through the utilization of the *Cumulative Index to Nursing and Allied Health Literature* (*CINAHL*) an excellent-sounding article on a topic of special research interest. Indexes are generic; that is, they index articles in their area of specialization without regard to the holdings of a particular library. Just because the researcher finds an entry in the index for an article does not mean that his library owns the journal that carries that article. Many steps and much time will be saved if the researcher will check the holdings list to see if the library actually subscribes to the periodical in question and, equally important, if the subscription includes the date of the sought-after article. Without the information provided in the holdings list, the researcher is destined to waste valuable time by scurrying up and down the aisles of the Bound Periodicals Section looking for the treasure, which may not even be there.

The Bound Periodicals Section may be alphabetized or classified by subject, depending on the practice of the particular library. Some libraries may not shelve bound periodicals by themselves but interfile them on the shelves with the books.

In most U.S. libraries, bound periodicals stacks are open to the patron so that the researcher is allowed to search out the needed journal issue independently. In some libraries, however, the stacks are closed and the researcher must request that the journals be brought to him.

Although we will discuss this point later, it should be emphasized here that the researcher must write down legibly the complete bibliographic information before beginning the search for needed materials. Frustration compounds confusion when the researcher must return again and again to the original reference in the index to get yet more information about the notation that should have been written down in its entirety at the outset.

The sad truth is that some researchers have only the faintest idea of what the Bound Periodicals Section is or how to use it. It constitutes yet another great gray bog of mystery and superstition and, therefore, is infrequently used, particularly by the undergraduate. Too often researchers presume on the basis of a quick perusal of only a few current periodicals in the Current Periodicals Section, or, even worse, a casual glance through the library catalog, that the library has nothing on the subject under consideration.

The Bound Periodicals Section of the library constitutes a secret treasury that can be opened only through the use of the indexes, but once the key is discovered, namely, how to use the indexes, that great treasury willingly offers up its holdings to the earnest researcher.

Reading a periodical. Unfortunately, inexperienced researchers too often pass over some of the added attractions in the periodical literature. In addition to finding the especially applicable article in the scholarly journal, the observant researcher will find even more. First, in some scholarly journals, the articles are preceded by a substantial and very helpful "abstract," a paragraph, often in bold or italic type, which summarizes the contents of the article. The abstract will indicate immediately to the researcher whether this particular article is going to be of value. Often the title is not exactly descriptive of the contest, but the abstract most definitely is. By reading the abstract, the researcher may save valuable time.

Furthermore, if a researcher is attempting to develop a topic by first preparing a research bibliography, an effective device is finding a crucial article in the periodical literature, turning to its conclusion, and finding there a well-developed bibliography already prepared by the scholar who wrote the article. Often, two or three such articles will turn up more bibliographical citations than a researcher can handle for a single research project. Otherwise, a researcher might spend hours wandering the aisles of the library "hoping" to find a bibliography on the topic at hand, never realizing that such bibliographies are there if he only knew where to look.

Indexes

Periodicals indexes are an indispensable category of reference works for the researcher of nursing and health sciences. Rather than spending hours browsing through journals at random—or even making "educated guesses"—trying to find material on the needed topic, the skilled researcher will turn to the indexes, wherein articles are categorized and arranged by subject. Though too numerous for a complete list here, we will give a brief description of the ones most valuable to the researcher of nursing and health sciences. We will include a sample entry for several of them in the illustrations. Some entries index periodicals and journals and others index other reference books. There are several basic indexes every researcher should know, most of which can be found in any library.

Many of these indexes are available in both paper and electronic format. Some contain citations only or citations plus abstracts, while others contain the full text of the original article. The scholar will want to inquire which indexes the library has and in which format.

An increasing number of indexes are now available in electronic format. Like their print counterparts, these indexes are not free and can generally be accessed through a library that has a subscription. In many cases, the online version has some decided advantages because it is often more current, contains a greater number of articles or citations, and often contains the full text of the articles. In some cases, while the index does not contain the full text of the article, it contains an electronic link to cited articles to which the library maintains subscription rights. In some cases, the electronic version of an index may contain an electronic link to a book that the library holds in electronic format.

Another advantage of the online indexes is that the scholar can often search multiple years in a single search, whereas print volumes are usually bound a year at a time and must be searched year by year. Some online indexes allow a search to be refined by narrowing the search to particular dates, a particular language or languages, or a specific journal or journals.

Because things change quickly in this area, no attempt is made here to be inclusive. As many of these indexes are published by the H.W. Wilson Company, the researcher may want to check the Wilson Web site at http://www.hwwilson.com for the latest information on a particular index and its content.

Annual Review of Nursing Research (New York: Springer, 1984–) is a valuable source of information on what nursing has accomplished in the field of research. Each

Bibliographic Index

A Cumulative Bibliography of Bibliographies

APRIL 2003

A

A-bomb *See* Atomic bomb
A.D.C. *See* Child welfare
Aberdeen (Scotland)
History
Aberdeen before 1800; a new history. Tuckwell Press 2002 p479-98
Ability, Social *See* Social skills
Abiogenesis *See* Life—Origin
Abnormal children *See* Exceptional children; Handicapped children
Abnormalities *See* Plants—Abnormalities
Abnormalities (Plants) *See* Plants—Abnormalities
Abnormalities in plants *See* Plants—Abnormalities
Abolition of slavery *See* Slavery
Aborigines *See* Indigenous peoples
Aborigines, American *See* Indians
Aborigines, Australian *See* Australian aborigines
Abortion
Myrsiades, Linda S. Splitting the baby; the culture of abortion in literature and law, rhetoric and cartoons. (Eruptions, v. 20) Lang, P. 2002 p175-98
Abortion, Induced *See* Abortion
Abravanel, Isaac, 1437-1508
By and about
Borodowski, Alfredo Fabio. Isaac Abravanel on miracles, creation, prophecy, and evil; the tension between medieval Jewish philosophy and biblical commentary. (Studies in biblical literature, v. 53) Lang, P. 2003 p219-33
Absence from work *See* Absenteeism (Labor)
Absent treatment *See* Mental healing
Absenteeism (Labor)
Cohen, A. The relationship between commitment forms and work outcomes: A comparison of three models. *Hum Relat* v53 no3 p414-17 Mr 2000
Dishon-Berkovits, M. and Koslowsky, M. Determinants of Employee Punctuality. *J Soc Psychol* v142 no6 p735-9 D 2002
Absolute differential calculus *See* Calculus of tensors
Abu Hamid Al-Ghazâli *See* Al-Ghazâli, 1058-1111
Abuse of animals *See* Animal welfare
Abuse of children *See* Child abuse
Abuse of husbands *See* Husband abuse
Abuse of substances *See* Substance abuse
Abuse of the aged *See* Aged—Abuse of
Abuse of wives *See* Wife abuse
Abused children
Psychology
Maughan, A. and Cicchetti, D. Impact of Child Maltreatment and Interadult Violence on Children's Emotion Regulation Abilities and Socioemotional Adjustment. *Child Dev* v73 no5 p1540-2 S/O 2002
Toth, S. L. and others. Relations Among Children's Perceptions of Maternal Behavior, Attributional Styles, and Behavioral Symptomatology in Maltreated Children. *J Abnorm Child Psychol* v30 no5 p499-501 O 2002
Abused family members *See* Victims of family violence
Abused women
Supriya, K. E. (Karudapuram Eachambadi). Shame and recovery; mapping identity in an Asian women's shelter. Lang, P. 2002 p265-76
Legal status, laws, etc.
Weldon, S. L. Beyond Bodies: Institutional Sources of Representation for Women in Democratic Policymaking. *J Polit* v64 no4 p1171-4 N 2002
Psychology
Carlson, B. E. and others. Intimate Partner Abuse and Mental Health: The Role of Social Support and Other Protective Factors. *Violence Against Women* v8 no6 p742-5 Je 2002
Hardesty, J. L. Separation Assault in the Context of Postdivorce Parenting: An Integrative Review of the Literature. *Violence Against Women* v8 no5 p621-5 My 2002
Swan, S. C. and Snow, D. L. Behavioral and Psychological Differences Among Abused Women Who Use Violence in Intimate Relationships. *Violence Against Women* v9 no1 p106-9 Ja 2003

Services for
Scott, E. K. and others. Dangerous Dependencies: The Intersection of Welfare Reform and Domestic Violence. *Gender Soc* v16 no6 p894-7 D 2002
Sullivan, C. M. and others. Findings From a Community-Based Program for Battered Women and Their Children. *J Interpers Violence* v17 no9 p933-5 S 2002
Abusing men *See* Abusive men
Abusing women *See* Abusive women
Abusive boyfriends *See* Abusive men
Abusive fathers *See* Abusive men
Abusive husbands *See* Abusive men
Abusive men
Hamberger, L. K. and Guse, C. E. Men's and Women's Use of Intimate Partner Violence in Clinical Samples. *Violence Against Women* v8 no11 p1327-31 N 2002
Counseling of
Augusta-Scott, T. and Dankwort, J. Partner Abuse Group Intervention: Lessons From Education and Narrative Therapy Approaches. *J Interpers Violence* v17 no7 p801-5 Jl 2002
Psychology
Augusta-Scott, T. and Dankwort, J. Partner Abuse Group Intervention: Lessons From Education and Narrative Therapy Approaches. *J Interpers Violence* v17 no7 p801-5 Jl 2002
Carr, J. L. and VanDeusen, K. M. The Relationship Between Family of Origin Violence and Dating Violence in College Men. *J Interpers Violence* v17 no6 p643-6 Je 2002
Rosen, L. N. and others. Intimate Partner Violence Among Married Male U.S. Army Soldiers: Ethnicity as a Factor in Self-Reported Perpetration and Victimization. *Violence Victims* v17 no5 p620-2 O 2002
Abusive wives *See* Abusive women
Abusive women
Dasgupta, S. D. A Framework for Understanding Women's Use of Nonlethal Violence in Intimate Heterosexual Relationships. *Violence Against Women* v8 no11 p1383-9 N 2002
Gilbert, P. R. Discourses of Female Violence and Societal Gender Stereotypes. *Violence Against Women* v8 no11 p1297-300 N 2002
Hamberger, L. K. and Guse, C. E. Men's and Women's Use of Intimate Partner Violence in Clinical Samples. *Violence Against Women* v8 no11 p1327-31 N 2002
Perilla, J. L. and others. A Working Analysis of Womens Use of Violence in the Context of Learning, Opportunity, and Choice. *Violence Against Women* v9 no1 p42-6 Ja 2003
Swan, S. C. and Snow, D. L. Behavioral and Psychological Differences Among Abused Women Who Use Violence in Intimate Relationships. *Violence Against Women* v9 no1 p106-9 Ja 2003
Academic achievement
Arnold, D. H. and others. Accelerating Math Development in Head Start Classrooms. *J Educ Psychol* v94 no4 p768-70 D 2002
Becker, B. E. and Luthar, S. S. Social-Emotional Factors Affecting Achievement Outcomes Among Disadvantaged Students: Closing the Achievement Gap. *Educ Psychol* v37 no4 p209-14 Fall 2002
Jeynes, W. H. The effects of Black and Hispanic 12th graders living in intact families and being religious on their academic achievement. *Urban Educ* v38 no1 p53-7 Ja 2003
Kim, K. and Rohner, R. P. Parental Warmth, Control, and Involvement in Schooling: Predicting Academic Achievement Among Korean American Adolescents. *J Cross-Cult Psychol* v33 no2 p138-40 Mr 2002
Li, J. A Cultural Model of Learning: Chinese "Heart and Mind for Wanting to Learn". *J Cross-Cult Psychol* v33 no3 p266-9 My 2002
Luthar, S. S. and Becker, B. E. Privileged but Pressured? A Study of Affluent Youth. *Child Dev* v73 no5 p1607-10 S/O 2002
Marsh, H. W. and Kleitman, S. Extracurricular school activities: the good, the bad, and the nonlinear. *Harv Educ Rev* v72 no4 p509-11 Wint 2002
Marzano, Robert J. What works in schools; translating research into action. Association for Supervision & Curriculum Development 2003 p193-207

Figure 4.1A   Sample page from *Bibliographic Index* print

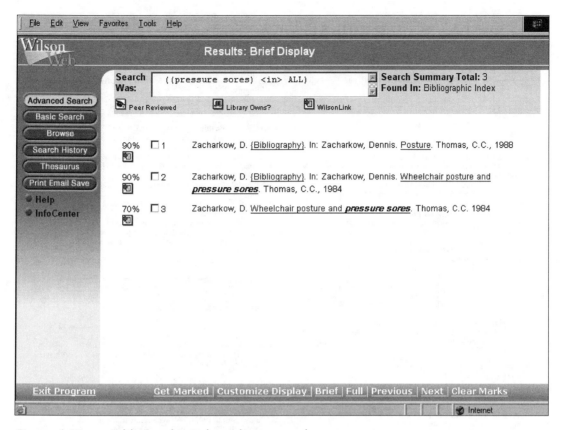

Figure 4.1B   *Bibliographic Index* online screenshot

volume presents a systematic review of all available research on specific topics in nursing. Beginning with Volume 18, each volume will have a more specific focus. Each volume will continue to have one or two chapters of general interest to nursing research.

Bibliographic Index, from H. W. Wilson Company, Bronx, NY, provides students and researchers with a useful tool to aid them in selecting information for their projects. It is a subject index to bibliographies in English and foreign languages that are found in current books, pamphlets, or periodicals. The *Bibliographic Index* covers most areas in which bibliographies are compiled and offers an indication of recent scholarship and new developments in many fields. Some 50,000 Monographs (books) and more than 2,800 periodicals are examined annually for material to be included in the index. To be listed, a bibliography must contain more than 50 citations. A sample entry from the print index is given in Figure 4.1A. It is now also available online (see Figure 4.1B).

Biography Index, from H.W. Wilson, is a guide to the location of biographical materials found in the books, pamphlets, and more than 3,000 periodicals appearing in

SEPTEMBER 2001–AUGUST 2002

50 Cent (Musician), American rap musician
Binelli, M. No. 1 With a Bullet [50 Cent] *Roll Stone* no915 p31-2 F 6 2003
Tyrangiel, J. Rap's Newest Target [50 Cent] por *Time* v161 no7 p68 F 17 2003

A

Aaliyah, 1979-2001, American singer
Farley, Christopher John. Aaliyah; more than a woman. MTV Bks./Pocket Bks. 2001 199p il por
Aaron, Didier, 1923-, French antique dealer
Mason, B. S. Reflections on a ™Golden Eye∫. il *Art Auction* v25 no1 p42-4 Ja 2003
Aaron, Hank, 1934-, baseball player
The Scribner encyclopedia of American lives, The 1960s, v1; William L. O'Neill, volume editor. Scribner 2003 p1-3 bibl il por
Aaron, Henry *See* Aaron, Hank, 1934-
Aaron, HervÇ, antique dealer
Mason, B. S. Reflections on a ™Golden Eye∫. il *Art Auction* v25 no1 p42-4 Ja 2003
Abate, Anne K., American professor of communications
Interviews
Anne K. Abate [Candidate for SLA director] por *Inf Outlook* v7 no1 p34 Ja 2003
Abbas, Mahmoud, 1935-, Palestinian political leader
Bennet, J. Israel Kills a Top Hamas Leader; Arafat Promotes Critic of Uprising. il map por *N Y Times (Late N Y Ed)* p1, 8 Mr 9 2003
Abbe, Cleveland, 1838-1916, meteorologist
Oakes, Elizabeth. A to Z of STS scientists. Facts on File 2002 p1-3 bibl il por
Abbot, Rufus, American fashion publicist
Marriage
Berk, S. His English Rose [Wedding of C. Rutherford and R. Abbott] il por *InStyle* v10 no2 p239 F 2003
Abdelhak, Sherif, foundation official
Galinski, T. Abdelhak reconsidered. il *Mod Healthcare* v32 no44 p30 N 4 2002
Abdi, Abbas, Iranian newspaper editor and former revolutionary
Trials, litigation, etc.
Iranian justice: A very strange confession. por *Economist* v366 p39 Ja 11 2003
Abdullah, Shadi, Jordanian Al Qaeda informer
Butler, D. and Van Natta, D., Jr. A Qaeda Informer Helps Investigators Trace Group's Trail. il *N Y Times (Late N Y Ed)* p A1, A12 F 17 2003
Aberconway, Charles Melville McLaren, 3rd Baron, 1913-2003, English shipbuilder
Obituary
N Y Times (Late N Y Ed) por p B7 F 8 2003
Aberdeen, George Hamilton Gordon, Earl of, 1784-1860, British statesman
Cavendish, R. Lord Aberdeen Becomes Prime Minister December 19th, 1852. *Hist Today* v52 no12 p52-3 D 2002
Abernathy, Kathleen, regulatory official
Spaniolo, J. D. Opening Luncheon Remarks [Communications Law and Policy Symposium] *Law Rev Mich State Univ Detroit Coll Law* v2002 no3 p755 Fall 2002
Abeshouse, Adam, recording producer
Singer, M. Play It Again [A. Abeshouse, founder of the Classical Recording Foundation] il *New Yorker* v78 no39 p38, 40 D 16 2002
See also
Abraham, Lynne D., d. 2002, public relations consultant and breast cancer patient
Obituary
N Y Times (Late N Y Ed) p66 D 15 2002
Abrams, Creighton Williams, 1914-1974, general
The Scribner encyclopedia of American lives, The 1960s, v1; William L. O'Neill, volume editor. Scribner 2003 p3-5 bibl il por

Abrasha, Dutch jeweler
Gans, J. C. Studio Visit: Abrasha. il por *Metalsmith* v22 no5 p18-19 Fall 2002
Abruzzese, Joseph, 1947-, television executive
Higgins, J. M. Abruzzese goes over to the cable side. por *Broadcast Cable* v132 no43 p14 O 21 2002
McClellan, S. Discovery Challenge. por *Broadcast Cable* v132 no47 p18, 20 N 18 2002
Abu Bakar Bashir *See* Bashir, Abu Bakar
Abu Hamid Al-Ghazālī *See* Al-Ghazālī, 1058-1111
Abu Kishek, Munir, Palestinian boxer
Bennett, J. In Nablus, Strife Dims Dreams and Daily Life. il map por *N Y Times (Late N Y Ed)* p1, 6 D 29 2002
Abu Mazin *See* Abbas, Mahmoud, 1935-
Abu Nidal, Palestinian terrorist
Obituary
N Y Times Mag por p48-9 D 29 2002
See also
Abzug, Bella, congresswoman and feminist
The Scribner encyclopedia of American lives, The 1960s, v1; William L. O'Neill, volume editor. Scribner 2003 p5-6 bibl il por
See also
See also
Ackerman, Thomas P., 1947-, meteorologist
Oakes, Elizabeth. A to Z of STS scientists. Facts on File 2002 p3-4 bibl il por
Acord, James L., Jr., sculptor
Interviews
James Acord: Atomic artist. il por *Nucl News* v45 no12 p50-8 N 2002
Acord, Lance, cinematographer
Hart, H. Writer's Block. il por *Am Cinematogr* v83 no12 p66-8, 70, 72-3 D 2002
See also
Adam, Christopher T., chemical engineer
Interviews
Johnson, P. K. Newsmaker: An Interview with Christopher T. Adam. por *Int J Powder Metall* v38 no8 p15-16 N/D 2002
Adams, Ansel, 1902-1984, American photographer
Croke, B. The Visual West: Moran, Jackson, Adams. il *Am Spectator* v36 no1 p60-2 Ja/F 2003
Adams, Charles Francis, 1807-1886, congressman and diplomat
Brookhiser, Richard. America's first dynasty; the Adamses, 1735-1918. A Large print ed Thorndike Press 2002 456p bibl
Adams, Cindy, gossip columnist
Adams, C. Puppy Love [Excerpt from The Gift of Jazzy] por *Good Housekeep* v236 no2 p58-60, 62, 66 F 2003
Interviews
Wayne, G. Cindy Adams puts on the dog. por *Vanity Fair* no510 p114 F 2003
Adams, Douglas, 1952-2001, English science fiction writer and satirist
Philips, Deborah. Douglas Adams. (In British fantasy and science-fiction writers since 1960. Gale Group 2002 p3-7) bibl il por
Adams, Henry, 1838-1918, historian
Brookhiser, Richard. America's first dynasty; the Adamses, 1735-1918. A Large print ed Thorndike Press 2002 456p bibl
Biographical works
O'Rourke, P. J. Third Person Singular [book, The Education of Henry Adams] il *Atl Mon (1993)* v290 no5 p34-7 D 2002
Political and social views
O'Rourke, P. J. Third Person Singular [book, The Education of Henry Adams] il *Atl Mon (1993)* v290 no5 p34-7 D 2002
Adams, John, 1735-1826, American president
Brookhiser, Richard. America's first dynasty; the Adamses, 1735-1918. A Large print ed Thorndike Press 2002 456p bibl
Adams, John Quincy, 1767-1848, American president
Brookhiser, Richard. America's first dynasty; the Adamses, 1735-1918. A Large print ed Thorndike Press 2002 456p bibl

Figure 4.2A   Page from print *Biography Index*

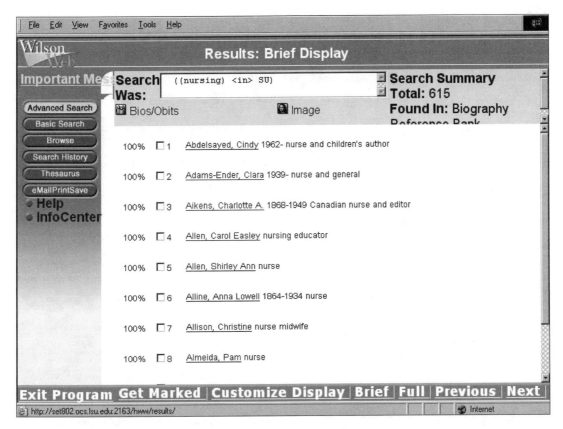

File   Edit   View   Favorites   Tools   Help

Wilson
Web

Results: Brief Display

Important Mes... **Search Was:**   ((nursing) <in> SU)

Advanced Search
Basic Search
Browse
Search History
Thesaurus
eMailPrintSave
● **Help**
● **InfoCenter**

Bios/Obits   Image

Search Summary
Total: 615
Found In: Biography
Reference Bank

100% ☐1   Abdelsayed, Cindy 1962- nurse and children's author

100% ☐2   Adams-Ender, Clara 1939- nurse and general

100% ☐3   Aikens, Charlotte A. 1868-1949 Canadian nurse and editor

100% ☐4   Allen, Carol Easley nursing educator

100% ☐5   Allen, Shirley Ann nurse

100% ☐6   Alline, Anna Lowell 1864-1934 nurse

100% ☐7   Allison, Christine nurse midwife

100% ☐8   Almeida, Pam nurse

Exit Program Get Marked | Customize Display | Brief | Full | Previous | Next

http://set802.ocs.lsu.edu:2163/hww/results/   Internet

Figure 4.2B   Screenshot from *Wilson Biographies Online*

other Wilson indexes. Access to all types of biographical writing from primary and secondary sources is provided. These include autobiographies, bibliographies, critical studies, literature, letters, memoirs, pictorial works, and poetry. More than 2,500 books of individual and collective biography are indexed annually. Approximately 1,600 records are added monthly. The obituaries in the *New York Times* are regularly included. Incidental materials found in prefaces, chapters, and bibliographies of otherwise nonbiographical works are considered important sources. *Biography Index* consists of a main alphabetical entry by last name of the subject, with a cross-reference index by profession. The index contains a checklist of composite books analyzed. Portraits and other illustrations are noted. Entries include a wide variety of people from antiquity to the present and are chosen from all fields and nationalities. The print index is updated quarterly and the online version is updated monthly. It is available online in several versions, including versions with extensive full text availability. Figure 4.2A gives a sample entry from the print index, while Figure 4.2B shows an entry from the online index.

BOOK REVIEW DIGEST

APRIL 2003

(Subject and Title Index follows the review listings)

A

THE ABBREVIATED PSALTER OF THE VENERABLE BEDE; translated by Gerald M. Browne. 92p $18 2001 Eerdmans
    264.028   1. Psalters
    ISBN 0-8028-3919-3   LC 2001-40533

SUMMARY: This is a translation of "the abbreviated psalter of the Venerable Bede (died 735), one of the earliest devotional manuals. . . . [Browne] thinks that this kind of book was meant both as a manual of prayer and a summary of the meaning of each individual psalm." (Commonweal)

REVIEW: *Commonweal* v129 no18 p30 O 25 2002. Lawrence S. Cunningham (50-500w)
"I am always on the lookout for good resources on the Psalms. The psalter is at the heart of Christian prayer, and I use it when teaching about prayer in the classroom. . . . [Bede] spent his whole life as a monk. He probably knew the psalter by heart; it was the core of the monastic office. Bede had the fine idea of excerpting a verse or two from each of the Psalms, presumably indicating the essence of each, and compiling them into a single book. . . . As I worked through this short but handsomely produced volume, I realized it might be used as an instructional tool. . . . It would also make a wonderful gift to someone who loves the Psalms."

ABEL, RICHARD, 1941-, ed. The Sounds of early cinema. See The Sounds of early cinema

ACKERMAN, BRUCE A., ed. Bush v. Gore. See Bush v. Gore

ADKINS, LESLEY. The keys of Egypt; the obsession to decipher Egyptian hieroglyphs; [by] Lesley and Roy Adkins. 335p il maps $25 2000 HarperCollins Publishers
    493   1. Egyptian language—Writing, Hieroglyphic 2. Champollion, Jean François, 1790-1832
    ISBN 0-06-019439-1   LC 00-38320

SUMMARY: The authors tell the story of French Egyptologist and decipherer Jean-François Champollion. "When Napoleon invaded Egypt in 1798, his troops [found] . . . countless ruins covered with hieroglyphs—remnants of a language lost in time. Egyptomania spread throughout Europe with their return, and the quest to decipher the hieroglyphs began in earnest. . . . In rural France, Champollion, the . . . son of an impoverished bookseller, became obsessed with breaking the code of the ancient Egyptians. . . . In 1812, Champollion made the decisive breakthrough, beating his closest rival, English physician Thomas Young, to the prize and becoming the first person to be able to read the ancient Egyptian language in well over a thousand years." (Publisher's note) Index.

REVIEW: *London Rev Books* v24 no18 p11-12 S 19 2002. John Sturrock (501-1000w)
"Champollion's is the life-story told in The Keys of Egypt. It is told efficiently and in much detail, though by authors who don't have any great feel for the hazards and shifts contingent on a life lived first in Napoleonic—Champollion was born in 1790—and then Restoration France; who see a need to locate the Louvre every time it is mentioned; and who sink to a new low

in asinine anglicisation by turning the Ecole Normale into the Normal School. The book's one real fault, however, is strategic: inflexibly chronological as it is, it introduces the technicalities of the decipherment piecemeal, according to how well Champollion was doing, with the result that his epochal achievement is harder to follow than it need have been."

ADKINS, ROY. The keys of Egypt. See Adkins, L.

ADLER, NANCI, 1963-. The Gulag survivor; beyond the Soviet system. 290p $34.95 2001 Transaction Pubs.
    365   1. Political prisoners—Soviet Union 2. Political persecution—Soviet Union—Psychological aspects 3. Concentration camps—Soviet Union
    ISBN 0-7658-0071-3   LC 2001-41595

SUMMARY: This study is based on interviews with former Soviet political prisoners. Adler focused "her inquiry first on the official and legal aspects of rehabilitation, readaptation, and what she calls 'resocialization' into Soviet society. . . . The stress of resuming their lives, while simultaneously keeping silent about what had happened to them, compounded the physical and psychological damage which Soviet prisoners had already suffered. As a result, Adler writes, many victims developed 'concentration camp syndrome'—persistent anxiety and depression continuing for many years after release. . . . Others were unable to shake off the camp culture, unable to readjust to a 'normal' life." (NY Rev Books) Index.

REVIEW: *N Y Rev Books* v49 no16 p40-2 O 24 2002. Anne Applebaum (501-1000w)
"Adler's conclusions, for the most part, are grimly predictable. Yet there remains one aspect of the rehabilitation of Soviet prisoners for which she cannot quite account: the undeniable enthusiasm, even happiness, with which returnees rejoined the Communist Party. . . . Nanci Adler grapples with this conundrum—'allegiance to a belief system can have deep non-rational roots,' she writes—but is mostly interested in other things. To Catherine Merridale [Night of Stone: Death and Memory in Twentieth-Century Russia], on the other hand, the issue is fundamental, lying at the heart of her own investigation into Soviet history."

ADORNO, THEODOR W. (THEODOR WIESENGRUND), 1903-1969. Beethoven; the philosophy of music: fragments and texts; edited by Rolf Tiedemann; translated by Edmund Jephcott. 268p il $40.50; pa $17.95 2002 Stanford Univ. Press
    780.92   1. Music—Philosophy and aesthetics 2. Beethoven, Ludwig van, 1770-1827
    ISBN 0-8047-3515-8; 0-8047-4711-3 (pa)
    LC 98-60570

SUMMARY: "For a great part of his life, Adorno worked at a book on Beethoven. He did not succeed in finishing it, but left a mass of notes, now published, along with a few articles, [including] . . . two on Beethoven's Missa Solemnis and on his late style." (N Y Rev Books) Indexes.

REVIEW: *N Y Rev Books* v49 no16 p59-66 O 24 2002. Charles Rosen (1000+w)
"The essay on the late style—by which Adorno meant the late quartets and late sonatas as well as the Diabelli Variations and the Ninth Symphony—reveals both Adorno's strength and his limitations. . . . Adorno's perceptive observation about the conventional formulae in the late style is illuminating, but he fails to understand that Beethoven had become by then simply more laconic, more economical. . . . What causes him to misrepresent the character of the late work is his too easy identification of convention with objectivity and original expression with subjectivity. . . . He is hamstrung by the Romantic view that genius consists chiefly in breaking the rules."

Figure 4.3A   Sample page from print *Book Review Digest Plus*

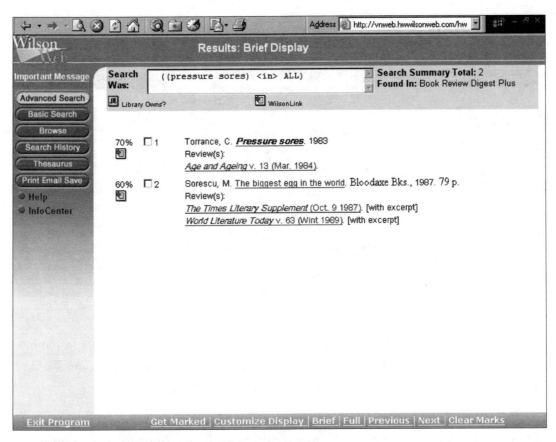

Figure 4.3B   *Book Review Digest Plus* online screenshot

Book Review Digest, from H.W. Wilson, cites and provides short excerpts of reviews of current English-language fiction and nonfiction books from more than 100 American, British, and Canadian periodicals. Reviews are added for 8,000-plus books of adult and juvenile fiction and nonfiction in the humanities, social sciences, and general sciences each year. To qualify for inclusion, a book must have been either published or distributed in the United States or Canada. Each book is listed alphabetically in *Book Review Digest* by main entry, usually the author. Title, bibliographical information, descriptive information, review excerpts, and citations follow. This main section is followed by a subject and title index. The print version has quarterly cumulations and a permanent bound annual cumulation. The online version, called *Book Review Digest Plus,* is updated weekly and dramatically expands the scope of the printed version. It encompasses more than a million reviews, covering more than 700,000 books. The inclusion of excerpts from reviews often provides the needed information without making it necessary for the researcher to locate the actual review

PRESCRIPTIVE AUTHORITY

Nurse prescribing: week 3. Nurses' influence on GPs' prescribing (Burns D) (CEU, research) **NURS TIMES** 2002 Oct 22-28; 98(43): 41-2 (6 ref)

Special focus. Nurse prescribing: week 4. Extended prescribing powers: three views (Burns D et al) (CEU) **NURS TIMES** 2002 Oct 29-Nov 4; 98(44): 37-8 (3ref)

Perspectives on prescribing: pioneers' narratives and advice (Hales A) (quesionnaire/scale, research, tables/charts) **PERSPECT PSYCHIATR CARE** 2002 Jul-Sep; 38(3); 79-88 (6 ref)

Prescriber's diary: a practice nurse view of nurse prescribing training. The tools of the trade... (Lawrie J) (anecdote) **PRACT NURSE** 2002 Nov 8; 24(8): 74

Prescriber's diary: a practice nurse view of nurse prescribing training. In it for the long haul... (Searie D) (anecdote) **PRACT NURS** 2002 Nov 22; 24(9): 66

Prescriber's diary: a practice nurse view of nurse prescribing training. Life in the fast lane... (Lawrie J) (anecdote) **PRACT NURSE** 2002 Dec 13; 24(10): 50

LEGISLATION AND JURISPRUDENCE

Advocacy in practice. Advocating for NPs — go and do likewise (Edmunds M) **NURSE PRACT** 2003 Feb; 28(2): 56

Nurses fail to disclose decubitus ulcers: punitive damages awarded: case on point: NME Properties, Inc v. Rudich, 2003 WL 289415 So.2d — FL (Tammelleo AD) (legal cases) **NURS LAW REGAN REP** 2003 Feb; 43(9): [2]

Pressure ulcer prevention and management in palliative care (Hampton S) (pictorial) **NURSE NURSE** 2003 Jan; 3(2): 24-6 (30 ref)

Pressure ulcers: part 1 (Fletcher J) (pictorial, teaching materials) **PROF NURSE** 2002 Dec; 18(4): 2p (4 ref)

Pressure ulcers: part 1 (Fletcher J) (pictorial) **PROF NURSE** 2002 Dec; 18(4): Professional Nurse Explaining Wounds Card Series: 9: 2p (4 ref)

CLASSIFICATION

Classification systems. Pressure ulcer classification: defining early skin damage (Russell L) (review, tables/charts) **BR J NURS** 2002 Sep; 11(16): Tissue Viability Suppl: S33-4, S36, S38+ (45 ref)

DRUG THERAPY

Nutrition Q&A. Vitamin C and pressure ulcers (Collins N) (questions and answers, tables/charts) **ADV SKIN WOUND CARE** 2002 Jul-Aug; 15(4): 186, 188 (8 ref)

Comment. What is the evidence for specific pressure-reducing mattresses? (Russell L) **BR J NURS** 2002 Nov; 11(20): Tissue Viability Supplement: S5 (8ref)

Product focus. DEEP CELL PRIME: preventing and healing pressure ulcers (Gray D) (pictorial, review, tables/charts) **BR J NURS** 2002 Nov; 11(20): Tissue Viability Supplement: S44, S46-8 (31 ref)

Estimation of the economic cost of pressure ulcers prevention in a hospital unit (Pancorbo Hidalgo PL et al) (pictorial, research, table/charts) **GEROKOMOS** 2002; 13(3): 164-71 (29 ref) [Spanish]

Knowledge and use of the recommendations about prevention and treatment of pressure ulcers in health centers from Andalucía (García Fernández FP et al) (research, tables/charts) **GEROKOMOS** 2002; 13(4): 214-22 (14 ref) [Spanish]

Contempo updates: linking evidence and experience. Pressure ulcer prevention and management (Lyder CH) (tables/charts) **JAMA** 2003 Jan 8; 289(2): 223-6 (30 ref)

Staff involvement in skin care leads to smooth success (Mahnke K et al) **NURS SPECTRUM (CHICAGO ILLINOIS INDIANA)** 2002 Sep 23; 15(19): 15

Figure 4.4A   Sample excerpt from print *CINAHL*

itself. Reviews of textbooks, government publications, and technical books in the law and sciences are excluded. Figure 4.3A shows an example of the print version and Figure 4.3B shows the online version of *Book Review Digest Plus*.

Book Review Index, from Gale, Farmington Hills, Michigan, is similar in scope and purpose to *Book Review Digest*. The major difference is that *Book Review Index* gives only citations for the reviews and does not include excerpts.

Cumulative Index to Nursing and Allied Health Literature (*CINAHL*; Glendale, CA: Glendale Adventist Medical Center, 1977–) provides authoritative coverage of the literature related to nursing and allied health professions. *CINAHL* began publication in 1977 and is updated monthly. It predominantly indexes articles in English but does index some selected foreign-language journals along with the publications of the American Nurses Association (ANA) and the National League for Nursing (NLN). Primary journals are indexed from the following allied health fields: cardiopulmonary technology, emergency service, health education, medical/laboratory technology, medical records, nutrition, occupational therapy, physical therapy, radiologic technology, respiratory therapy, and social service in healthcare.

Other journals selectively indexed cover the areas of consumer health, biomedicine, and health sciences librarianship. More than 1,200 journals are regularly indexed. The index also provides access to healthcare books, book chapters, pamphlets, nursing dissertations, selected conference proceedings, standards of professional practice, nurse

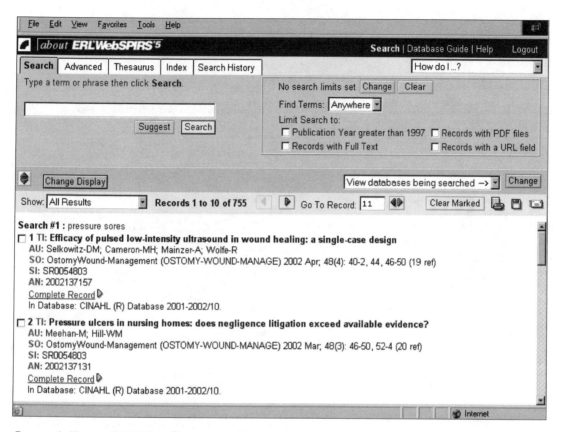

Figure 4.4B   *CINAHL* online screenshot

practice acts, critical paths, research instruments, educational software, and audiovisuals in nursing.

More than 10,000 *CINAHL* subject headings provide specific access to Nursing and Allied Health Literature citations. Approximately 70 percent of *CINAHL* headings also appear in the MEDLINE database. *CINAHL* supplements these headings with 2,000-plus terms designed specifically for nursing and allied health. Figure 4.4A shows a page from the print index. Figure 4.4B gives a sample entry from the online version.

Current Book Review Citations (1976–1982), from H.W. Wilson, is an index of book reviews appearing in more than 1,200 periodicals between 1976 and 1982. It provides users with a guide to recent reviews of fiction and nonfiction books found in both book-reviewing periodicals and subject periodicals. *Current Book Review Citations* assists readers in locating critical evaluations from a wide variety of periodicals during those years. All the major fields of intellectual and scientific pursuits are encompassed:

EDUCATION INDEX

APRIL 2003

3-D television *See* Television, Stereoscopic
16mm films *See* Motion picture films
403(b) plan
Stock market has some retirees rethinking their plans. il *Am Teach* v87 no4 p7 D 2002/Ja 2003

A

A levels (Advanced) examination
Lack of support blamed for fiasco. W. Mansell. *Times Educ Suppl* no4517 p14 Ja 31 2003
AAAS *See* American Association for the Advancement of Science
AACTE *See* American Association of Colleges for Teacher Education
Aanrud, Kelly
Just listen to us. *Engl J* v92 no3 p13-14 Ja 2003
AASA *See* American Association of School Administrators
AAU *See* Association of American Universities
AAUP *See* American Association of University Professors
Abbreviations
See also
Signs and symbols
ABE (Adult basic education) *See* Basic education
Abecedarian Project
Investing in Preschool. G. W. Bracey. il *Am Sch Board J* v190 no1 p32-5 Ja 2003
Ability
See also
Creative ability
Mathematical ability
Motor ability
Physical ability
Success
Ability and achievement
See also
Student achievements
Underachievement
The contribution of general and specific cognitive abilities to reading achievement. M. L. Vanderwood and others. bibl graph *Learn Individ Differ* v13 no2 p159-88 2001
The wrong responses to a very difficult item: a comparison of high-scoring and low-scoring examinees. D. Cairns and others. tab *Int J Math Educ Sci Technol* v33 no6 p839-42 N/D 2002
Ability grouping
Elementary schools
Primaries dig heels in over setting. B. Passmore. *Times Educ Suppl* no4518 p4 F 7 2003
Hong Kong
Learning and motivation of Chinese students in Hong Kong: a longitudinal study of contextual influences on students' achievement orientation and performance. F. Salili and M. K. Lai. bibl graph tab *Psychol Sch* v40 no1 p51-70 Ja 2003
Abingdon (Va.)
Public schools
Challenging Gifted Students [A. Linwood Holton Governor's School] S. Rapp. *Sci Teach* v70 no1 p10 Ja 2003
Able, Graham, 1947-
Attitudes, opinions, etc.
HMC leader calls for end to awards for rich. C. Canovan. *Times Educ Suppl* no4513 p3 Ja 3 2003
To serve them by deserts. C. Canovan. por *Times Educ Suppl* no4513 p10 Ja 3 2003
Abnormal psychology *See* Pathological psychology
Abolitionists
See also
Underground railroad
Aborigines, Australian *See* Australian aborigines
Aborigines, Tasmanian *See* Tasmanian aborigines
Aboud, Frances E.
The Formation of In-Group Favoritism and Out-Group Prejudice in Young Children: Are They Distinct Attitudes? bibl tab *Dev Psychol* v39 no1 p48-60 Ja 2003

Abram, Suzanne
The Americans with Disabilities Act in Higher Education: The Plight of Disabled Faculty. bibl f *J Law Educ* v32 no1 p1-20 Ja 2003
Abrams, Nathan
It's time to rock the lecture boat. il *Times Higher Educ Suppl* no1572 p29 Ja 17 2003
Abramson, Ilene
A Haven for Homeless Kids. *SLJ* v49 no1 p41 Ja 2003
Absences
See also
Attendance
Truancy
Absolute value
Examining Continuity, Partial Derivatives and Differentiability with Cylindrical Coordinates. T. C. McMillan. graph il *Coll Math J* v34 no1 p11-14 Ja 2003
Abstinence (Sexual) *See* Chastity
Abstract algebra
Problems, exercises, etc.
On positive functions with positive derivatives. D. E. Dobbs. *Int J Math Educ Sci Technol* v33 no6 p895-8 N/D 2002
Sets of Sets: A Cognitive Obstacle. L. Brenton and T. G. Edwards. bibl f il *Coll Math J* v34 no1 p31-8 Ja 2003
Abstract art
See also
Abstract expressionism
Abstract expressionism
Cave Kids: Pecos River-Style Art. S. T. Clark. il *Arts Act* v132 no5 p32-3, 51 Ja 2003
Abstraction
See also
Categorization (Psychology)
Mental representation
Abused children
See also
Child abuse survivors
Sexually abused children
Catch-up growth assessment in long-term physically neglected and emotionally abused preschool age male children. G. Oliván. bibl tab *Child Abuse Neglect* v27 no1 p103-8 Ja 2003
Mental health
Psychological correlates of physical abuse in Hong Kong Chinese adolescents. J. T. F. Lau and others. bibl tab *Child Abuse Neglect* v27 no1 p63-75 Ja 2003
ACA *See* Academic Co-operation Association
Academe (Periodical)
Indexes
Index to Academe. *Academe* v88 no6 p79-84 N/D 2002
Academic achievement *See* Student achievements
Academic advisement *See* Educational guidance
Academic Co-operation Association
Study finds little reality in English horror stories. D. Jobbins. *Times Higher Educ Suppl* no1571 p12 Ja 10 2003
Academic credits *See* Credits and credit systems
Academic deans *See* Deans
Academic degrees *See* Degrees, Academic
Academic dissertations
Digital travail on the way to a dissertation. A. Samuel. *Chron Higher Educ* v49 no19 p B5 Ja 17 2003 supp
Great Expectations: Tips for a Successful Working Relationship with Your Thesis Advisor. M. W. Tanner. *Coll Stud J* v36 no4 p635-44 D 2002
Repository company creates online-submissions process for dissertations. F. Olsen. *Chron Higher Educ* v49 no20 p A30 Ja 24 2003
Evaluation
Toward principled practice in evaluation: learning from instructors' dilemmas in evaluating graduate students. N. Sabar. bibl *Stud Educ Eval* v28 no4 p329-45 2002
Preparation
Navigating in unknown waters: proposing, collecting data, and writing a qualitative dissertation. C. Bencich and others. *Coll Compos Commun* v54 no2 p289-306 D 2002
Academic environment *See* Organizational climate (in education)

Figure 4.5A   Sample page from *Education Index*

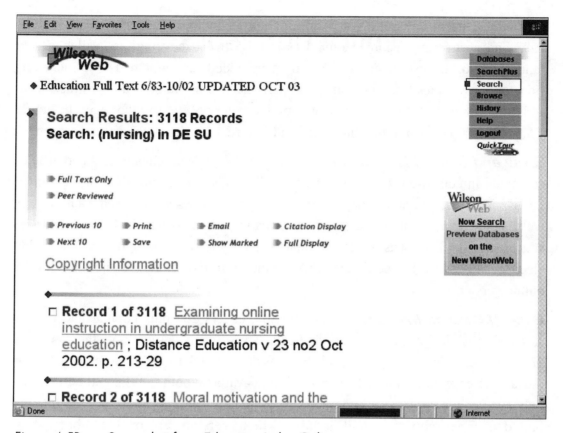

Figure 4.5B   Screenshot from *Education Index Online*

business, education, the humanities, law, the social sciences, and pure and applied sciences. Part I of *Current Book Review Citations* is the "Author Index." All book reviews are entered by the name of the author of the book reviewed. The title and the date of publication of the book are given, followed by the name of the periodical in which the review appeared with its volume number, date, and page numbers. The name of the reviewer is included if available. Part II is the "Title Index." When a title is used as the main entry, the full bibliographic information is to be found in the "Author Index" with a "see" reference from the entry in the Title Index.

Education Index, from H.W. Wilson, covers approximately 600 core English-language periodicals, books, and yearbooks published in the U.S. and elsewhere on a wide range of contemporary education issues such as multicultural education, religious education, student counseling, and information technology. Indexing began in June 1983 and abstracting began in June 1984, and full text coverage is available from January 1996. Approximately 3,000 records are added each month. The full text version contains articles from more than 500 periodicals plus citations and abstracts from additional journals. Abstracts are from approximately 50 to 150 words each. Figure 4.5A shows a page from the print index and Figure 4.5B shows the online version.

Essay and General Literature Index, from H.W. Wilson, cites essays and articles contained in collections of essays and miscellaneous works published in the United States, Great Britain, and Canada. More than 300 volumes are indexed each year, as well as more than 20 annuals and serial publications. Approximately 4,000 records are added annually. The focus is on the humanities and social sciences. It is now available electronically as well. (See Figure 4.6A for the print version and Figure 4.6B for the online version.)

General Science Index, from H.W. Wilson, covers 200-plus popular and professional English-language science periodicals. The "Science" section of the *New York Times* is also included. Citations and abstracts extend back to 1984. More than 50 periodicals are covered in full text since 1995. It is available both in print and online. The online version is available as an index only, as an index plus abstracts, or with full text included. The scholar should inquire which version his or her library has. Approximately 5,000 records are added monthly. Figure 4.7A shows a page from the print version of the *General Science Index*. Figure 4.7B shows the online version of *Applied Science and Technology Index*.

Humanities Index. This H.W. Wilson index covers more than 500 English-language periodicals in the humanities. Among the disciplines included are literature and language, history, philosophy, archeology, classical studies, folklore, and religion and theology. Indexing and abstracting covers back to 1984. More than 175 periodicals are covered in full text from 1995 to date; 3,000-plus entries are added monthly. Abstracts range from approximately 50 to 150 words each. It is available both in print and online. The online version is available as an index only, as an index plus abstracts, or with full text included. The scholar should inquire which version his or her library has. In 2003, Wilson introduced *Humanities Retrospective,* indexing periodicals back to 1907. Figure 4.8A shows a page from the print index and Figure 4.8B shows the online index.

Index Medicus is NLM's (National Library of Medicine) bibliographic index of citations and abstracts from 4,600 journals published in the United States and more than 70 other countries. This literature has been judged most useful to *Index Medicus* users

Essay and General Literature Index

2002

9 to 5 (Motion picture) *See* Nine to five (Motion picture)

10 things I hate about you (Motion picture)
Burt, R. T(e)en things I hate about girlene Shakesploitation flicks in the late 1990s; or, Not-so-fast times at Shakespeare High. (*In* Spectacular Shakespeare; ed. by C. Lehmann and L. S. Starks p205-32)

11th Amendment *See* United States. Constitution. 11th Amendment

60s (Twentieth century decade) *See* Nineteen sixties

1960s *See* Nineteen sixties

A

A-bomb *See* Atomic bomb

A. E. *See* Russell, George William, 1867-1935

A.I. (Motion picture)
O'Brien, G. The mechanical child. (*In* O'Brien, G. Castaways of the image planet p235-39)

Aaron, Hank, 1934-
About individual works
I had a hammer
Altherr, T. L. For the record and lives that mattered: American baseball autobiographies. (*In* The Cooperstown symposium on baseball and American culture, 2001 p231-45)

Aaron, Henry *See* Aaron, Hank, 1934-

Aarons, Victoria
A kind of vigilance: tropic suspension in Bernard Malamud's fiction. (*In* The Magic worlds of Bernard Malamud; ed. by E. Avery p175-86)

Abbate, Carolyn
In search of opera
Contents
Debussy's phantom sounds
Magic flute, nocturnal sun
Metempsychotic Wagner
Orpheus. One last performance
Outside the tomb

Abbott, Andrew Delano
The disciplines and the future. (*In* The Future of the city of intellect; ed. by S. Brint p205-30)

Ability
See also Intellect

Ablow, Rachel
Labors of love: the sympathetic subjects of David Copperfield. (*In* Dickens studies annual, v31 p23-46)

Abolition of slavery *See* Slavery

Abortion
Barro, R. J. Abortion and crime. (*In* Barro, R. J. Nothing is sacred p73-77)

Abrahamson, Edward A.
Zen Buddhism and The assistant: a grocery as a training monastery. (*In* The Magic worlds of Bernard Malamud; ed. by E. Avery p69-86)

Abruzzi (Italy)
Ginzburg, N. Winter in the Abruzzi. (*In* Ginzburg, N. A place to live p35-40)

Abstraction
See also Concepts

Abuse of substances *See* Substance abuse

Abuse of wives *See* Wife abuse

Abused wives
See also Wife abuse

Accident law
See also Torts

Accountability, Criminal *See* Criminal liability

Acculturation
Suárez-Orozco, C. Psychocultural factors in the adaptation of immigrant youth: gendered responses. (*In* Women, gender, and human rights; ed. by M. Agosín p170-88)

Achilles (Greek mythology) in literature
Edwards, M. W. Homer I: poetry and speech. (*In* Edwards, M. W. Sound, sense, and rhythm p1-37)

Achinstein, Sharon
Samson Agonistes and the politics of memory. (*In* Altering eyes; edited by M. R. Kelley & J. Wittreich p168-91)

Acker, Kathy, 1948-1997
About
Cooley, N. Painful bodies: Kathy Acker's last texts. (*In* We who love to be astonished; ed. by L. Hinton and C. Hogue p193-202)
Harryman, C. Rules and restraints in women's experimental writing. (*In* We who love to be astonished; ed. by L. Hinton and C. Hogue p116-24)

About individual works
Empire of the senseless
Conte, J. M. Discipline and anarchy: disrupted codes in Kathy Acker's Empire of the senseless. (*In* Conte, J. M. Design and debris p54-74)

In memorian to identity
Duvall, J. N. Postmodern Yoknapatawpha: William Faulkner as usable past. (*In* Faulkner and postmodernism; ed. by J.N. Duvall & A. J. Abadie p39-56)

Ackroyd, Peter
About individual works
T. S. Eliot
Ricks, C. Peter Ackroyd: T. S. Eliot. (*In* Ricks, C. Reviewery p59-68)

Acorn, Milton, 1923-1986
About
Waterston, E. Burns, Acorn, and the rivers of song. (*In* Waterston, E. Rapt in plaid p12-42)

Figure 4.6A   Sample page from *Essay and General Literature Index*

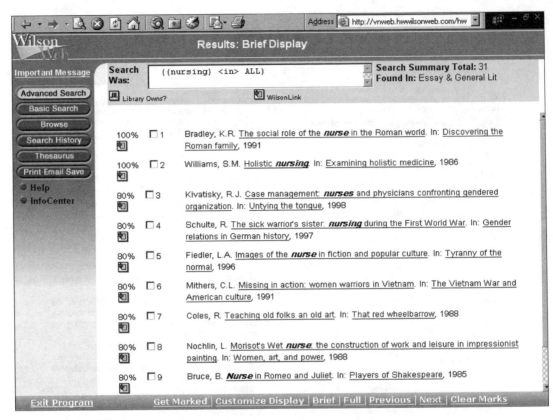

Figure 4.6B   *Essay and General Literature* online screenshot

by a group of distinguished physicians, medical editors, and medical librarians. Materials selected for inclusion are indexed by highly trained literature analysts. Monthly issues consist of two volumes: Part 1 Subject A–P and Part 2 Subject Q–Z, Authors and Bibliography of Medical Reviews. The cumulated contents of the twelve monthly issues comprise the annual *Cumulated Index Medicus*, which is now discontinued. The subject scope of *Index Medicus* is biomedicine and health, broadly defined to encompass those areas of the life sciences, behavioral sciences, chemical sciences, and bioengineering needed by health professionals and others engaged in basic research and clinical care, public health, health policy development, or related educational activities. It also covers nursing, dentistry, veterinary medicine, pharmacy, allied health, and preclinical sciences. The majority of publications covered in *Index Medicus* are scholarly journals; a small number of newspapers, magazines, and newsletters are also included. Figure 4.9A is a sample excerpt from the print index. Figure 4.9B shows the online version.

GENERAL SCIENCE INDEX

APRIL 2003

1/f noise *See* Random noise
3-D imaging *See* Three dimensional imaging
3-D models *See* Three dimensional models
5-HT receptors *See* Serotonin receptors
5-Hydroxytryptamine *See* Serotonin
5-Hydroxytryptamine inhibitors *See* Serotonin uptake inhibitors
18th century *See* Eighteenth century

A

Abalones
Using Spatially Explicit Data to Evaluate Marine Protected Areas for Abalone in Southern California. L. Rogers-Bennett and others. bibl graph map tab *Conserv Biol* v16 no5 p1308-17 O 2002
ABC transporters
Regulation
Analysis of a DtxR-Like Metalloregulatory Protein, MntR, from Corynebacterium diphtheriae That Controls Expression of an ABC Metal Transporter by an Mn^{2+}-Dependent Mechanism. M. P. Schmitt. bibl diag graph il tab *J Bacteriol* v184 no24 p6882-92 D 2002
Abciximab
Long-Term Survival Benefit After Use of Abciximab? G. B. Huffman. *Am Fam Phys* v66 no10 p1985 N 15 2002
Abdomen
See also
Pelvis
Abdominal fat distribution and peripheral and hepatic insulin resistance in type 2 diabetes mellitus. Y. Miyazaki and others. bibl graph il tab *Am J Physiol* v283 no6 p E1135-E1143 D 2002 pt1
Tumors
Fish
A Three-Year Retrospective Study of Abdominal Tumors in Zebrafish Maintained in an Aquatic Laboratory Animal Facility. R. Smolowitz and others. bibl il *Biol Bull* v203 no2 p265-6 O 2002
Aberrant tissue *See* Choristoma
Abnormal enzymes *See* Abnormal proteins
Abnormal peptides *See* Abnormal proteins
Abnormal proteins
Additions and Corrections: Isolation and Structure Elucidation of Chlorofusin, a Novel p53-MDM2 Antagonist from a Fusarium sp. *J Am Chem Soc* v124 no48 p14503 D 4 2002
Abortion pill RU-486 *See* Mifepristone
Abscission (Botany)
Abscission, Dehiscence, and Other Cell Separation Processes. J. A. Roberts and others. bibl il *Annu Rev Plant Biol* v53 p131-58 2002
Absorption
See also
Packed columns
Kinetics
Study of the Effects of Particle-Phase Carbon on the Gas/Particle Partitioning of Semivolatile Organic Compounds in the Atmosphere Using Controlled Field Experiments. B. T. Mader and J. F. Pankow. bibl graph tab *Environ Sci Technol* v36 no23 p5218-28 D 1 2002
Absorption (Physiology)
See also
Biosorption
Intestinal absorption
Kidneys—Physiology
Absorption of soils *See* Soil absorption and adsorption
Absorption spectroscopy
See also
Atomic absorption spectroscopy
Abstraction reactions
Hydrogen Atom Abstraction by a Chromium(IV) Oxo Complex Derived from O_2. K. Qin and others. bibl il *J Am Chem Soc* v124 no47 p14008-9 N 27 2002
Abused women
Domestic Violence—Medieval and Modern [Images of health] E. Fee and others. bibl f il *Am J Public Health* v92 no12 p1908 D 2002
Abyssinian wolf *See* Simien jackal
Acceleration due to gravity *See* Gravity and gravitation
Accelerators (Particles)
See also
Electron accelerators
Synchrotrons
Access control
See also subhead Access control under the following subjects
Internet
Accident prevention *See* Safety devices and measures
Accidents
See also
Falls (Accidents)
First aid in illness and injury
Home accidents
Traffic accidents
Wounds
Nonfatal Sports- and Recreation-Related Injuries Treated in Emergency Departments—United States, July 2000-June 2001. *JAMA* v288 no16 p1977-9 O 23-30 2002
Accidents, Industrial *See* Industrial accidents
Acclimation
Increased lipogenesis in isolated hepatocytes from cold-acclimated ducklings. E. Bedu and others. bibl graph tab *Am J Physiol* v283 no5 p R1245-R1253 N 2002 pt2
Acclimatization
Similar carbohydrate but enhanced lactate utilization during exercise after 9 wk of acclimatization to 5,620 m. G. Van Hall and others. bibl graph tab *Am J Physiol* v283 no6 p E1203-E1213 D 2002 pt1
Accreditation of hospitals *See* Hospitals—Accreditation
Accretion (Astrophysics)
A Classical Nova, V2487 Opd 1998, Seen in X-rays before and after its Explosion. M. Hernanz and G. Sala. bibl f graph *Science* v298 p393-5 O 11 2002
Weird Black-Hole Topography Proposed. J. Winters. *Discover* v24 no1 p72 Ja 2003
Accumulation, Biological *See* Bioaccumulation
ACE inhibitors *See* Angiotensin-converting enzyme inhibitors
Acetaminophen
Iterative High-Throughput Polymorphism Studies on Acetaminophen and an Experimentally Derived Structure for Form III. M. L. Peterson and others. bibl il *J Am Chem Soc* v124 no37 p10958-9 S 18 2002
Risk Assessment of an Acetaminophen Baiting Program for Chemical Control of Brown Tree Snakes on Guam: Evaluation of Baits, Snake Residues, and Potential Primary and Secondary Hazards. J. J. Johnston and others. bibl il *Environ Sci Technol* v36 no17 p3827-33 S 1 2002
Acetates
Derivatives
Trifluoroacetylsulfenyl Trifluoroacetate, $CF_3C(O)–S–O–C(O)CF_3$, a Novel Compound with a Symmetrically Substituted S–O Bond: Synthesis, Spectroscopic Characterization, and Quantum Chemical Calculations. S. E. Ulic and others. bibl f graph il tab *Inorg Chem* v41 no22 p5699-705 N 4 2002
Oxidation
Kinetic and Mechanistic Study of the Atmospheric Oxidation by OH Radicals of Allyl Acetate. B. Picquet-Varrault and others. bibl diag graph tab *Environ Sci Technol* v36 no19 p4081-6 O 1 2002
Acetone bodies *See* Ketone bodies
Acetonitriles
Probing Transport and Microheterogeneous Solvent Structure in Acetonitrile-Water Mixtures and Reversed-Phase Chromatographic Media by NMR Quadrupole Relaxation. E. D. Dawson and S. L. Wallen. bibl il *J Am Chem Soc* v124 no47 p14210-20 N 27 2002

Figure 4.7A Sample page from print *General Science Index*

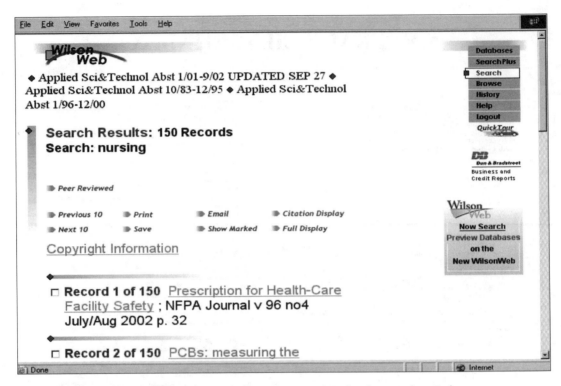

Figure 4.7B   Screenshot from *Applied Science and Technology Index Online*

Index to U.S. Government Periodicals, (1970–1987) provides a subject and author approach to 120 periodicals issued by various agencies of the federal government. Published quarterly from 1970 to 1987, it is particularly useful for the social sciences for those years and, for an extensive search, should be used with the *Social Science Index*.

MEDLINE is NLM's (National Library of Medicine) bibliographic index of citations and abstracts from 4,600 health science journals published in the U.S. and more than 70 other countries. While the coverage is worldwide, the abstracts are all in English. This electronic index covers fields of medicine, nursing, dentistry, veterinary medicine, the healthcare system, the preclinical sciences, and some other areas of the life sciences. The database uses the NLM MeSH (Medical Subject Heading) indexing system and tree structures, allowing the user to display major subject headings and related sub-headings at a glance, with a thesaurus available for locating all related terms. Coverage is 1966 to date and back to 1964 at OLDMEDLINE. NLM provides free access to MEDLINE through a Web-based retrieval system, PubMed. PubMed contains links to full-text articles at participating publishers' Web sites. MEDLINE is also available from many online vendors, such as SilverPlatter/Ovid WebSPIRS (see Figure 4.9C) and EBSCO. It is updated weekly at NLM and monthly by most vendors.

HUMANITIES INDEX

MARCH 2003

8 Women [film] See Motion picture reviews—Single works
20th century See Twentieth century
24 hour party people (Motion picture)
Dream Factory: 24 Hour Party People. N. Young. *Crit Q* v44 no3 p80-7 Aut 2002
28 Days Later . . . [film] See Motion picture reviews—Single works
1848 revolutions See Europe—History—1848-1849
1930s See Nineteen thirties
1951 See Nineteen fifty-one
1960s See Nineteen sixties
1970s See Nineteen seventies
1990s See Nineteen nineties
2000 See Two thousand (Year)

A

À la recherche du temps perdu (Novel) See Proust, Marcel, 1871-1922—Works—À la recherche du temps perdu
A priori
Deeply Contingent A Priori Knowledge. J. Hawthorne. *Philos Phenom Res* v65 no2 p247-69 S 2002
À toi pour toujours (Drama) See Tremblay, Michel, 1942-—Works—À toi pour toujours
Aaron, Jonathan
Elsewhere [poem] *Times Lit Suppl* no5196 p23 N 1 2002
AAVE See Black English
Abba (Musical group)
Two-Tier Theatre? What does the Mirvishes' success mean for Canadian theatre? M. Hays. *Can Theatre Rev* no111 p100-1 Summ 2002
Abbasids
Competitive Hagiography in Biographies of al-Awzā S and Sufyān al-ThawrS. S. C. Judd. *J Am Orient Soc* v122 no1 p25-37 Ja/Mr 2002
The Redemption of Umayyad Memory by the ᶜAbbāsids [with appendix] T. El-Hibri. *J Near East Stud* v61 no4 p241-65 O 2002
ʾAbd al-Raḥmān I, Caliph of Cordova, 731-787 or 8
about
Competitive Hagiography in Biographies of al-Awzā S and Sufyān al-ThawrS. S. C. Judd. *J Am Orient Soc* v122 no1 p25-37 Ja/Mr 2002
Abe, Kōbō, 1924-1993
The Boom in Science Fiction (1962); tr. by C. Bolton. *Sci-Fict Stud* v29 pt3 p342-9 N 2002
Science Fiction, the Unnameable (1966); tr. by T. Schnellbächer. *Sci-Fict Stud* v29 pt3 p349-50 N 2002
about
Two Essays on Science Fiction [Introduction to essays by Kobo Abe] C. Bolton. *Sci-Fict Stud* v29 pt3 p340-1 N 2002
Abeillé, Anne, and Godard, Danièle
The Syntactic Structure of French Auxiliaries. bibl diag *Language* v78 no3 p404-52 S 2002
Aberdeen, George Hamilton Gordon, Earl of, 1784-1860
about
Lord Aberdeen Becomes Prime Minister: December 19th, 1852. R. Cavendish. *Hist Today* v52 no12 p52-3 D 2002
Ability
See also
Intellect
Leadership
Abolition of slavery See Antislavery movements
Abolitionist fiction See Slavery in literature
Abolitionists
The Banneker Literary Institute of Philadelphia: African American Intellectual Activism Before the War of the Slaveholders' Rebellion. T. Martin. bibl f *J Afr Am Hist* v87 p303-22 Summ 2002
Aboriginal peoples' first contact with Westerners See Indigenous peoples—Contact with Westerners
Aborigines See Indigenous peoples

Abortion
Ethical aspects
Abortion in the Tides of Culture. F. Mathewes-Green. *First Things* no128 p16-18 D 2002
Laws and regulations
United States
See also
Roe v. Wade
Religious aspects
Catholic Church
How Not To Overturn Roe v. Wade. P. B. Linton. *First Things* no127 p15-16 N 2002
United States
Abortion in the Tides of Culture. F. Mathewes-Green. *First Things* no128 p16-18 D 2002
Abortion in mass media
Abortion in the Tides of Culture. F. Mathewes-Green. *First Things* no128 p16-18 D 2002
Abouna [film] See Motion picture reviews—Single works
Abraham, Pearl, 1960-
If Only: Finding America in Hasidism. bibl f *Mich Q Rev* v41 no4 p527-33 Fall 2002
Abreaction See Catharsis
Absence in literature
The Aesthetics of Absence and the Scopophilic Text: Robert Penn Warren's "Meet Me in the Green Glen". A. Berger. bibl *Style* v36 no2 p308-27 Summ 2002
James as Jilter: Absenteeism in "Washington Square". C. Ozick. *Am Sch* v71 no4 p53-9 Aut 2002
Absolute, The
Three Ends of the Absolute: Schelling on Inhibition, Hölderlin on Separation, and Novalis on Density. D. F. Krell. bibl f *Res Phenomenol* v32 p60-85 2002
Absolute rights See Natural law
Absolute space See Space and time
Absolution
See also
Confession
Abstract, The See Abstraction
Abstract art
Abstraction and Aura. K. Broadfoot. bibl f il *South Atl Q* v101 no3 p459-78 Summ 2002
Caio Fonseca. P. Elley. il *Bomb* no81 p10-13 Fall 2002
What Was Abstract Art? (From the Point of View of Hegel). R. B. Pippin. *Crit Inq* v29 no1 p1-24 Fall 2002
Abstract photography
See also
Photomontage
Abstracting and indexing services
See also
Information systems
Abstraction
Front Porch. H. L. Watson. por *South Cult* v8 no3 p1-5 Fall 2002
Abstracts
See also subhead Abstracts under the following subjects
Philosophy
Absurd (Philosophy) in literature
Zazie Dans la Brousse. D. Jullien. *Rom Rev* v91 no3 p263-78 My 2000
Abuse of wives See Wife abuse
Academic dissertations
Bibliography
Dissertations in Women's History. J. Erlen. *J Women's Hist* v14 no3 p183-5 Aut 2002
Dissertations of Note. R. Fordyce. *Child Lit* v30 p245-60 2002
Doctoral Dissertations 2001-2002. *Rev Metaphys* v56 no1 p225-44 S 2002
A List of Dissertations. J. T. Schreier and M. Pehl. *West Hist Q* v33 no3 p343-8 Aut 2002
Recent Dissertations. *Am Indian Q* v25 no4 p651-3 Fall 2001
Recent Doctoral Dissertations in Church and State. S. E. Rosenbaum. *J Church State* v44 no3 p644-5 Summ 2002
Academic freedom
See also
Students—Legal status, laws, etc.

Figure 4.8A   Sample page from print *Humanities Index*

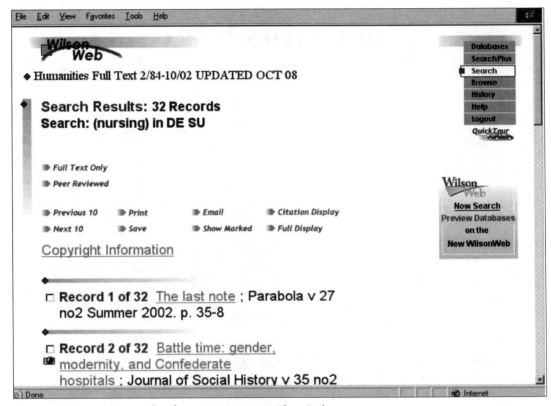

File   Edit   View   Favorites   Tools   Help

WilsonWeb

◆ Humanities Full Text 2/84-10/02 UPDATED OCT 08

Search Results: 32 Records
Search: (nursing) in DE SU

▸ Full Text Only
▸ Peer Reviewed

▸ Previous 10   ▸ Print   ▸ Email   ▸ Citation Display
▸ Next 10   ▸ Save   ▸ Show Marked ▸ Full Display

Copyright Information

☐ **Record 1 of 32** The last note ; Parabola v 27 no2 Summer 2002. p. 35-8

☐ **Record 2 of 32** Battle time: gender, modernity, and Confederate hospitals ; Journal of Social History v 35 no2

Databases
SearchPlus
Search
Browse
History
Help
Logout
QuickTour

Wilson Web
Now Search
Preview Databases
on the
New WilsonWeb

Done   Internet

Figure 4.8B   Screenshot from *Humanities Index Online*

Readers' Guide to Periodical Literature, from H.W. Wilson. This old standby from high school days is still useful to the university student and researcher of nursing and health sciences. Public libraries, which are often the only libraries available to nurses, may not have many of the previously mentioned titles, but most will have *Readers' Guide* (*RG*). Aimed at the general public, *RG* covers a broad spectrum of journals including several titles of interest to nurses and nursing students such as *Mayo Clinic Health Letter, Science News,* and *Psychology Today.* Articles from over 300 periodicals are indexed by author and subject, with entries for both located in a single alphabet. Each author and subject entry includes all the necessary bibliographic information to find the article cited: author's name, title of the article, title of the periodical, volume number, inclusive paging of the article, date of publication, and notations of illustrations, bibliographies, or other descriptive information. Book reviews are cited in a separate section. Approximately 7,000 items are added monthly. *RG* is issued monthly in print

DECISION MAKING

Parents' views of their children's participation in phase I oncology clinical trials. Deatrick JA, et al. **J Pediatr Oncol Nurs.** 2002 Jul-Aug; 19(4):114-21.

What is a moral dilemma and what would you do if you were faced with one? O'Neil JA. **J Pediatr Oncol Nurs.** 2002 Jul-Aug;19(4):145-7.

Decisions and revisions: the affective forecasting of changeable outcomes. Gilbert DT, et al. **J Pers Soc Psychol.** 2002 Apr;82(4):503-14.

Why Susie sells seashells by the seashore: implicit egotism and major life decisions. Pelham BW, et al. **J Pers Soc Psychol.** 2002 Apr;82(4)469-87.

Decision latitude and workload demand: implications for full and partial absenteeism. Zavala SK, et al. **J Public Health Policy.** 2002:23(3);344-61.

Racism in rape trials. Landwehr PH. et al. **J Soc Psychol.** 2002 Oct; 142(5):667-9.

Racial bias in decisions made by mock jurors evaluating a case of sexual harassment. Wuensch KL. et al. **J Soc Psychol.** 2002 Oct;142(5):587-600.

The importance of fracture pattern in guiding therapeutic decision-making in patients with hemorrhagic shock and pelvic ring disruptions. Eastridge BJ, et al. **J Trauma.** 2002 Sep;53(3):446-50; discussion 450-1.

Clinical judgment. Aronow WS. **Lancet.** 2002 Aug 24;360(9333):591.

Hormone replacement therapy to reduce cardiovascular risk: a concept whose time has passed? [editorial] Alpert MA. **South Med J.** 2002 Sep;95(9):959-61.

Lessons learned from the Women's Health Initiative study. [editorial] Hamdy RC. **South Med J.** 2002 Sep;95(9)951-2.

A gynecologist's view of hormone replacement therapy in light of the Women's Health Initiative. [editorial] Jelovsek FR. **South Med J.** 2002 Sep;95(9):955-7.

The rise and fall of hormone replacement therapy: oncologists' views. [editorial] Krishnan K. et al. **South Med J.** 2002 Sep;95(9):963-5.

After the Women's Health Initiative-what to tell our patients. [editorial] Muse K. **South Med J.** 2002 Sep;95(9)957-9.

Hormone replacement therapy and lipids: time to reconsider our options? [editorial] Peiris A, et al., **South Med J.** 2002 Sep;95(9)961-3.

Lessons from the Women's Health Initiative. [editorial] Watts NB. **South Med J.** 2002 Sep;95(9):952-5.

Management of solitary pulmonary nodules: how do thoracic computer tomograph and guided fine needle biopsy influence clinical decisions? Baldwin DR. et al. **Thorax.** 2002 Sep;57(9):817-22.

Odds ratio, relative risk, absolute risk reduction, and the number needed to treat—which of these should we use? Schechtman E. **Value Health.** 2002 Sep-Oct;5(5):430-5.

Cost-effectiveness of screening, surveillance, and primary prophylaxis strategies for esophageal varices. Arguedas MR, et al. **Am J Gastronterol.** 2002 Sep;97(9)2441-52.

Suspected inflammatory bowel disease—the clinical and economic impact of competing diagnostic strategies. Dubinsky MC. et al. **Am J Gastroenterol.** 2002 Sep;97(9):2333-42.

Comparison of two clinical prediction rules and implicit assessment among patients with suspected pulmonary embolism. Chagnon I. et al. Am J Med. 2002 Sep: 113(4):269-75. Comment in: **Am J Med.** 2002 Sep; 113(4):337-8.

Clinical prediction rules for the diagnosos of pulmonary embolism. [editorial] Ferreira G. et al. **Am J Med.** 2002 Sep;113(4):337-8. Comment on: **Am J Med.** 2002 Sep: 113(4):269-75.

Paraesophageal hernias: operation or observation? Stylopoulos N. et al. **Ann Surg.** 2002 Oct;236(4):492-500: discussion 500-1.

Bayesian estimation, simulation and uncertainty analysis: the cost-effectiveness of ganciclovir prophylaxis in liver transplantation. Vanness DJ, et al. **Health Econ.** 2002 Sep;11(6):551-66.

Treat or test first? Decision analysis of empirical antiviral treatment of influenza virus infection versus treatment based on rapid test results. Sintchenko V. et al. **J Clin Virol.** 2002 Jul;25(1):15-21.

A measure of agreement between clinicians and a computer-based decision support system for planning dental treatment. Kawahata N.et al. **J Dent Educ.** 2002 Sep;66(9):1031-7.

Figure 4.9A   Sample excerpt from *Index Medicus* in print

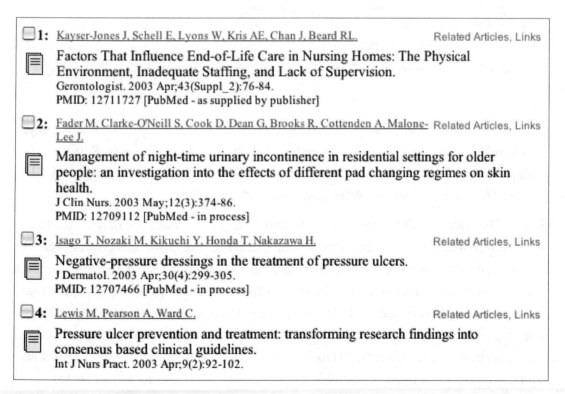

1: Kayser-Jones J, Schell E, Lyons W, Kris AE, Chan J, Beard RL.   Related Articles, Links

Factors That Influence End-of-Life Care in Nursing Homes: The Physical Environment, Inadequate Staffing, and Lack of Supervision.
Gerontologist. 2003 Apr;43(Suppl_2):76-84.
PMID: 12711727 [PubMed - as supplied by publisher]

2: Fader M, Clarke-O'Neill S, Cook D, Dean G, Brooks R, Cottenden A, Malone-Lee J.   Related Articles, Links

Management of night-time urinary incontinence in residential settings for older people: an investigation into the effects of different pad changing regimes on skin health.
J Clin Nurs. 2003 May;12(3):374-86.
PMID: 12709112 [PubMed - in process]

3: Isago T, Nozaki M, Kikuchi Y, Honda T, Nakazawa H.   Related Articles, Links

Negative-pressure dressings in the treatment of pressure ulcers.
J Dermatol. 2003 Apr;30(4):299-305.
PMID: 12707466 [PubMed - in process]

4: Lewis M, Pearson A, Ward C.   Related Articles, Links

Pressure ulcer prevention and treatment: transforming research findings into consensus based clinical guidelines.
Int J Nurs Pract. 2003 Apr;9(2):92-102.

Figure 4.9B   Online version of *Index Medicus* as provided by PubMed

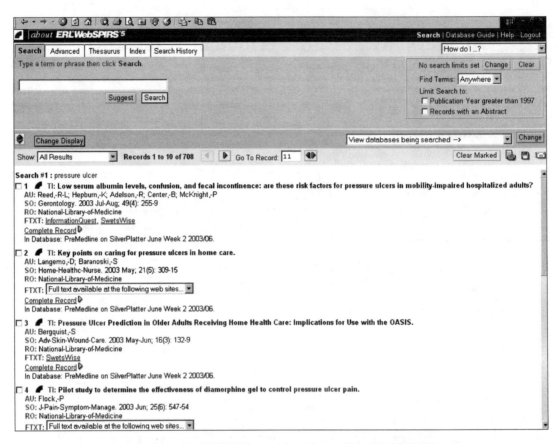

Figure 4.9C   Screenshot of MEDLINE from SilverPlatter/Ovid WebSPIRS

with annual cumulations. The print version dates back to 1900. *Readers' Guide* comes in several online versions, some including full text. *Readers' Guide Retrospective* (online) covers 1890–1982. A sample from the print version is given in Figure 4.10A. *Readers' Guide Full Text Online* is shown in Figure 4.10B.

Social Sciences Index, from H.W. Wilson. The *Social Sciences Index*, like many other Wilson indexes, comes in index, abstract, and full text formats. It covers over 500 English-language periodicals on topics such as anthropology, area studies, criminal justice, economics, international relations, political science, psychiatry, psychology, social work, and urban studies. Index coverage dates from 1983. Full text coverage of more than 150 periodicals dates back to 1995. Approximately 4,000 records are added each month. Abstracts run from 50 to 150 words each. It is available both in print and online. The online version is available as an index only, as an index plus abstracts, or with full text included. The scholar should inquire which version his library has. A

Readers' Guide to Periodical Literature

APRIL 2003

1-2-3 (Computer program) *See* Lotus 1-2-3 (Computer program)
3-D computer graphics
The human genome in 3D, at your fingertips. J. Bohannon. il *Science* v298 p737 O 25 2002
3-D displays
Getting Real. M. Alpert. il *Scientific American* v287 no6 p124-6 D 2002
3-D image processing
Getting Real. M. Alpert. il *Scientific American* v287 no6 p124-6 D 2002
3-D Imax motion pictures
Dawn in the Deep. R. A. Lutz. il map *National Geographic* v203 no2 p92-103 F 2003
3-D motion pictures
See also
3-D Imax motion pictures
3-D photography
History
A Virtual Reality Check. C. Baker. il *Wired* v11 no1 p68 Ja 2003
3-D television
Getting Real. M. Alpert. il *Scientific American* v287 no6 p124-6 D 2002
3-D video game machines
See also
PlayStation (Video game machine)
3-D video games
See also
Getaway (Game)
3deluxe (Firm)
Nuanced lighting at D'Fly in New York City casts a glow upon jewelry in a sleek setting fit for James Bond. L. B. French. il *Architectural Record* v190 no11 p238-40, 242 N 2002
3G mobile phone networks *See* Third generation wireless telecommunication
3SIXO (Firm)
3SIXO takes a brainy, multidisciplinary approach to the realm of design. W. Weathersby. il por *Architectural Record* v190 no12 p118-21 D 2002
4Runner (Automobile) *See* Toyota 4Runner (Automobile)
8 Mile [film] *See* Motion picture reviews—Single works
20/20 (Television program)
LA Lawman? [John Miller to leave 20/20] J. M. Robins. por *TV Guide* v51 no1 p45 Ja 4-10 2003
21 Club (New York, N.Y.: Restaurant)
'21' Pickup [The Upstairs at '21'] A. Platt. il *New York* v36 no4 p76-7 F 10 2003
24 (Television program)
What Makes 24 Tick? [Why is the Fox series 24 so popular?; cover story; special section] S. Malcom. il *TV Guide* v51 no1 p18-27 Ja 4-10 2003
25th hour (Motion picture)
Spike Lee [S. Lee talks about directing the film 25th Hour] J. Turturro. por *Interview* v33 no1 p70-1 F 2003
25th Hour [film] *See* Motion picture reviews—Single works
50 Cent (Musician)
about
No. 1 With a Bullet [50 Cent] M. Binelli. *Rolling Stone* no915 p31-2 F 6 2003
Rap's Newest Target [50 Cent] J. Tyrangiel. por *Time* v161 no7 p68 F 17 2003
100 days in the jungle (Television program)
Snakes and Ladders [The works of Canadian director S. Gunnarsson] B. D. Johnson. il por *Maclean's* v115 no50 p56-7 D 16 2002
401(k) plan
The Missing Link. M. B. Franklin. il tab *Kiplinger's Personal Finance* v57 no1 p78-80 Ja 2003
529 college savings plans *See* State college tuition savings plans
911 telephone numbers
Will your cell phone reach 911? il tab *Consumer Reports* v68 no2 p12-14 F 2003

A

A. B. Financing and Investments Inc.
Ethics
SEC Finds Miami Investment Firm Scammed Blacks. *Jet* v106 no2 p27 Ja 6 2003
A.I.: Artificial Intelligence [film] *See* Motion picture reviews—Single works
AAAS *See* American Association for the Advancement of Science
Aaliyah, 1979-2001
about
Aaliyah: I Care For U [sound recording] Reviews *Vibe* v11 no2 p136 F 2003. J. King
AAMC *See* Association of Art Museum Curators
Aarts, Michelle, and others
Treatment of ischemic brain damage by perturbing NMDA receptor-PSD-95 protein interactions. bibl f diag graph il *Science* v298 p846-50 O 25 2002
Abate, Frank
Nuclear. *The New York Times Magazine* p14 Ja 12 2003
Abbott Laboratories
Corrections & Clarifications [to Michael Arndt, An Ache at Amgen?] *Business Week* no3813 p14 D 23 2002
Abby (Television program)
Sydney Tamiia Poitier [Cover story] por *Jet* v103 no5 p58-60, 62 Ja 27 2003
ABC News
A Prime-Time Player [R. Arledge; H.Raines; editiorial] R. Rieder. *American Journalism Review* v25 no1 p6 Ja/F 2003
Abdel-Rahman, Omar
about
Tracing terror's roots. C. Ragavan. diag il por *U.S. News & World Report* v134 no6 p28-32 F 24 2003
Abdi, Abbas
about
Reformers at Bay in Iran. N. Thrupkaew. *The Nation* v276 no5 p6-7 F 10 2003
Abdomen
See also
Abdominal exercises
Abdominal exercises
Ab-solutely Necessary. E. Eyestone. il *Runner's World* v38 no1 p30 Ja 2003
The Core of the Matter. J. Purton. il *Runner's World* v38 no2 p38-40, 42-3 F 2003
Abdominal pain
The Health Problem Nobody's Talking About. L. Gottlieb. il *Glamour* v100 no11 {i.e. 101 no1} p54-5 Ja 2003
Abebooks (Web site)
Turning Old Books into Gold. K. MacQueen. il *Maclean's* v116 no4 p30-1 Ja 27 2003
Aberdeen, George Hamilton Gordon, Earl of, 1784-1860
about
Lord Aberdeen Becomes Prime Minister: December 19th, 1852. R. Cavendish. *History Today* v52 no12 p52-3 D 2002
Ability
See also
Creativity
Learning, Psychology of
Mathematical ability
Motor ability
Success
ABM (Anti-ballistic missile) system *See* Guided missiles—Defenses
Abolitionists
See also
Underground Railroad
Aborigines, Australian *See* Australian aborigines
Abortifacients
See also
Mifepristone
Abortion
See also
Partial-birth abortion
Saving black babies [Prolife movement targets black community] S. Blunt. *Christianity Today* v47 no2 p21-3 F 2003

Figure 4.10A   Sample page from print *Readers' Guide*

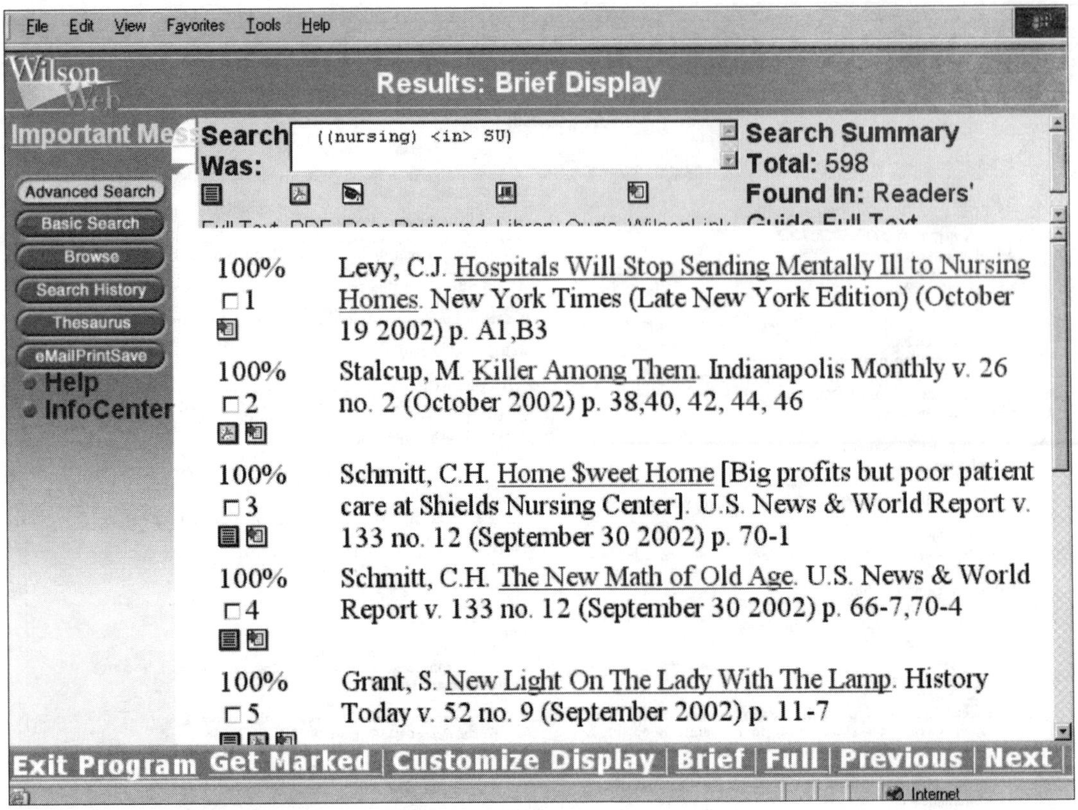

Figure 4.10B   Screenshot from *Readers' Guide*

sample of the print version is shown in Figure 4.11A and a sample from the online index is given in Figure 4.11B.

Vertical File Index, from H.W. Wilson, is a guide to pamphlets from many public and private sources, including businesses; federal, state, and local governments; not-for-profit organizations; think tanks; and small presses. Updated monthly, it indexes more than 3,000 sources each year. A sample page from the print index is shown in Figure 4.12.

Several of the previously mentioned indexes, and many others, are now available online. An increasing number of them are becoming available as CD-ROM products or via the World Wide Web and are more likely than ever to be found even in smaller libraries. Ask which indexes are available at your library or nearby libraries.

In addition to the previously mentioned indexes, some libraries subscribe to online services through one of several subscription services. Before beginning online research

SOCIAL SCIENCES INDEX

MARCH 2003

3G mobile phone networks *See* Third generation wireless tele-communication
24 hour party people (Motion picture)
A Party of One. J. Parker. il *Am Prospect* v13 no17 p40-1 S 23 2002
60 Plus Association
Drug Money. M. Goozner. por *Am Prospect* v13 no19 p12-13 O 21 2002
401(k) plan
Pension Overhaul Legislation Approved by House Ways and Means In Fight to Control the Issue. J. H. Davis. *CQ Wkly* v60 no11 p710 Mr 16 2002

A

AAPA *See* American Association of Physical Anthropologists
Aapico (Firm)
Fast Lane To Success. S. W. Crispin. por *Far East Econ Rev* v165 no36 p38-40 S 12 2002
AAPOR *See* American Association for Public Opinion Research
Abadi, Jacob
Algeria's Policy Toward Israel: Pragmatism and Rhetoric. bibl f *Middle East J* v56 no4 p616-41 Aut 2002
Israel's Quest for Normalization with Azerbaijan and the Muslim States of Central Asia. bibl f *J Third World Stud* v19 no2 p63-88 Fall 2002
Abadir, Karim, and Talmain, Gabriel
Aggregation, Persistence and Volatility in a Macro Model. bibl graph *Rev Econ Stud* v69 no4 p749-79 O 2002
Abadir, Karim A., and Paruolo, Paolo
Simple Robust Testing of Regression Hypotheses: A Comment. *Econometrica* v70 no5 p2097-9 S 2002
ABB Asea Brown Boveri Ltd.
All over? graph *Economist* v365 p56 O 26 2002
Abbott, Ann A.
Health Care Challenges Created by Substance Abuse: The Whole Is Definitely Bigger than the Sum of Its Parts. bibl *Health Soc Work* v27 no3 p162-5 Ag 2002
Abboud, A. Robert, and Minow, Newton N.
Advancing Peace in the Middle East: The Economic Path Out of Conflict. *Foreign Aff* v81 no5 p14-16 S/O 2002
ABC *See* American Broadcasting Companies, Inc.
ABC News
Network news coverage of school shootings. B. Maguire and others. bibl tab *Soc Sci J* v39 no3 p465-70 2002
Abdel-Khalek, Ahmed
(jt. auth) See Lester, David, and Abdel-Khalek, Ahmed
Abdel-Khalek, Ahmed, and Lester, David
Can personality predict suicidality? A study in two cultures. bibl tab *Int J Soc Psychiatry* v48 no3 p231-9 S 2002
Abdel-Khalek, Ahmed M.
Why Do We Fear Death? The Construction and Validation of the Reasons for Death Fear Scale. bibl tab *Death Stud* v26 no8 p669-80 O 2002
Abdo, Diya
Uncovering the Harem in the Classroom: Tania Kamal-Eldin's "Covered: The Hejab in Cairo, Egypt" and "Hollywood Harems" Within the Context of a Course on Arab Women Writers. bibl *Women's Stud Q* v30 no1/2 p227-38 Spr/Summ 2002
Abdo, Nahla
Women, war and peace: reflections from the Intifada. bibl *Women's Stud Int Forum* v25 no5 p585-93 S/O 2002
Abdomen
See also
Liver
Stomach
Size
Waist Circumference, Body Mass Index, and Risk for Stroke in Older People. D. K. Dey and others. bibl f tab *J Am Geriatr Soc* v50 no9 p1510-18 S 2002
Abduction
See also
Kidnapping

Abdullah Ahmad Badawi *See* Badawi, Abdullah Ahmad
Abdullin, M., and others
The "Pepsi Generation". graph tab *Russ Soc Sci Rev* v43 no5 p4-15 S/O 2002
Abe-Kim, Jennifer, and others
Predictors of Help Seeking for Emotional Distress Among Chinese Americans: Family Matters. bibl tab *J Consult Clin Psychol* v70 no5 p1186-90 O 2002
Abecassis, Maurissa, and others
Mutual Antipathies and Their Significance in Middle Childhood and Adolescence. bibl tab *Child Dev* v73 no5 p1543-56 S/O 2002
Abela, John R. Z., and others
An Examination of the Response Styles Theory of Depression in Third- and Seventh-Grade Children: A Short-Term Longitudinal Study. bibl tab *J Abnorm Child Psychol* v30 no5 p515-27 O 2002
Abelam (Papua New Guinea people)
Religion and mythology
Zero Hour: Reflecting Backward, Looking Forward. R. Scaglion. bibl *Ethnohistory* v47 no1 p227-40 Wint 2000
Ability
See also
Athletic ability
Creative ability
Executive ability
Gifted children
Mathematical ability
Motor ability
Musical ability
Spelling ability
Verbal ability
Effects of Situational Self-handicapping and State Self-confidence on the Physical Performance of Young Participants. T. A. Ryska. bibl graph tab *Psychol Rec* v52 no4 p461-78 Fall 2002
The Influence of Individual Versus Aggregate Social Comparison and the Presence of Others on Self-Evaluations. J. T. Buckingham and M. D. Alicke. bibl graph tab *J Pers Soc Psychol* v83 no5 p1117-30 N 2002
Unrealistic Optimism and Perceived Control: Role of Personal Competence. J. Fernández-Castro and others. tab *Psychol Rep* v91 no2 p431-5 O 2002
Rating
Children's Competence and Value Beliefs From Childhood Through Adolescence: Growth Trajectories in Two Male-Sex-Typed Domains. J. A. Fredricks and J. S. Eccles. bibl graph tab *Dev Psychol* v38 no4 p519-33 Jl 2002
Ability, Influence of age on
See also
Age and memory
Cognition—Age factors
Ability, Musical *See* Musical ability
Ability grouping in education
See also
Gifted children—Education
Sociodemographic Diversity, Correlated Achievement, and De Facto Tracking. S. R. Lucas and M. Berends. bibl graph tab *Sociol Educ* v75 no4 p328-48 O 2002
Ability tests
See also
Achievement tests
Ball aptitude battery
Motor ability tests
Abizadeh, Arash
Does Liberal Democracy Presuppose a Cultural Nation? Four Arguments. bibl *Am Polit Sci Rev* v96 no3 p495-509 S 2002
Ablaza, Gerardo
Interviews
Cellular Dreams. J. Hookway. *Far East Econ Rev* v165 no35 p62 S 5 2002
ABM Treaty (1972) *See* Anti-Ballistic Missile Treaty (1972)
ABN AMRO Bank NV
In and out. D. Shirreff. *Economist* v364 p survey9 S 14 2002
Abnormal psychology *See* Psychology, Pathological
Abnormalities
See also
Brain—Abnormalities

Figure 4.11A   Sample page from *Social Sciences Index*

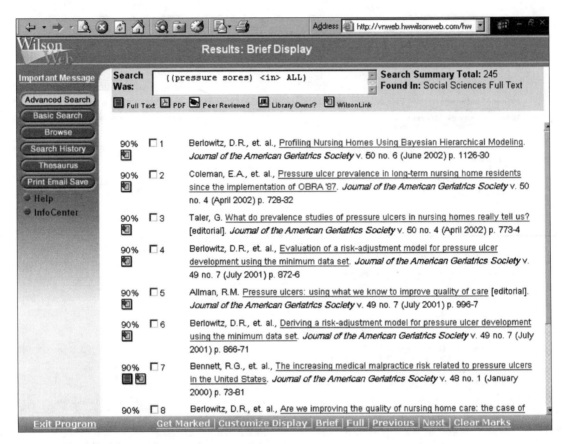

Figure 4.11B   *Social Sciences Full Text* online screenshot

through one of the vendors, the researcher should understand something about how charges are incurred, as searching online can be quite expensive. See Chapter 5 for more detail on how these charges are calculated.

Before you are scared off by the thought of paying hundreds of dollars to find a few articles, remember that the librarian is skilled at performing this type of search—some librarians more than others—so make sure you choose one who is skilled. An expert searcher can conduct a search and produce a list of relevant articles in just a few seconds or minutes. (Two minutes spent in a $300 per-hour database is only $10.)

It is for this reason that the librarian will often ask you to fill out one or more forms outlining your search and the desired results as carefully as possible. He will often ask you the maximum you want to spend and the number of citations you want to retrieve.

The reason for an online search is that it may be tailored to your needs much more exactly than a manual search. For example, you may be interested only in research that was published in the German language between 1983 and 1985. An online search will

VERTICAL FILE INDEX

MARCH 2003

A

Abortion
Laws and regulations
See also Abortion—Laws and regulations in Part 3
United States
Statistics
Induced abortion. (Facts in brief) 2p chart fig 2003 Alan Guttmacher Inst., 120 Wall St., New York, NY 10005 single copy free; multiple copies 25¢ ea; order or download at
http://www.agi-usa.org/
This fact sheet reports statistics on abortions in the U.S. Among other information, it reports that 49% of pregnancies are unintentional, that almost half of unintentional pregnancies are ended with abortions, and that increased use of emergency contraception has led to drops in abortion rates.

Abortion, Spontaneous *See* Miscarriage
Administrative assistants
Administrative assistant. (G-1-23) 4p col il 2003 Vocational Biogs. Inc., Box 31, Sauk Centre, MN 56378-0031 $5 plus 10% postage & handling ($1 minimum); send payment with order
This pamphlet describes the work of a woman who acts as a liaison between executives and customers and does secretarial work for a company. Includes information on job requirements and education needed.

Adolescence
See also
Youth
Adolescent crime *See* Juvenile delinquents and delinquency
Adult education and libraries *See* Libraries and adult education
Affirmative action
See also Affirmative action in Part 3
Afghanistan
History
Anti-terrorist operations, 2001- —Reconstruction
From Paris to Bonn; lessons for Afghanistan from the Cambodian transition, by Catharin E. Dalpino. (Working pa #14) 48p 2002 Asia Foundation, 465 California St., 14th Floor, San Francisco, CA 94104 single copy free; order or download at
http://www.asiafoundation.org/publications/
This paper suggests that people working to reconstruct Afghanistan would do well to look to the experience of Cambodia, still repairing the damage done by a regime that tried to destroy all preceding law and culture.

Africa
See also
AIDS (Disease) and children—Africa
Age and employment
See also
Child labor
Aged
Drug use
Aging, medicines and alcohol. [PHD882] 6p col il 2001 Natl. Clearinghouse for Alcohol & Drug Inf., Box 2345, Rockville, MD 20847-2345 free; toll-free no for ordering: 800-729-6686 (voice), 800-487-4889 (hearing impaired); enter title to order or download at
http://store.health.org/catalog/
This pamphlet explains that as people age their bodies respond differently to alcohol and medications, identifies signs that may indicate an alcohol or medication-related problem, and lists precautions to take with medications.
Medical care
Evaluation
Healthcare cost-effectiveness analysis for older patients; using cataract surgery and breast cancer treatment data, by Arash Naeim. (Dissertation RGSD-168) 166p charts col charts col figs tables 2002 Rand Corp., Publs. Dept., 1700 Main St., Box 2138, Santa Monica, CA 90407-2138 single copy free; order by e-mail at order@rand.org; enter rept. no. to order at
http://www.rand.org/Abstracts
This book discusses the general issue of evaluating medical treatments' cost effectiveness and the particular cases of immediate surgery versus watchful waiting for developing cataracts and hormonal versus combined chemical and hormonal adjuvant anti-cancer treatment in the aged.
Nutrition
Nutrition after fifty; tips and recipes. 36p il 2002 Am. Inst. for Cancer Res., Publs. Dept., 1759 R St. NW, Washington, DC 20009 single copy free; toll-free no for ordering: 800-843-8114; order or view at
http://www.aicr.org/cpublications.html
This booklet advises middle-aged people on good eating habits and nutrition. Recipes are included.

Agriculture
See also
Sustainable agriculture
AIDS (Disease) and children
HIV/AIDS and children affected by armed conflict. 3p il 2002 UNICEF, Programme Publs., 12-G, 3 UN Plaza, New York, NY 10017 single copy free; order or download at
http://www.unicef.org/infores/pubsdate.htm
This pamphlet reports that wars spread AIDS very quickly, and that children, who have least responsibility for the wars, are often both infected and orphaned in the accompanying plagues.
Statistics
Children on the brink 2002; a joint report on orphan estimates and program strategies. 36p chart figs il maps tables 2002 UNICEF, Programme Publs., 12-G, 3 UN Plaza, New York, NY 10017 single copy free; order or download at
http://www.unicef.org/infores/pubstitle.htm
This pamphlet provides statistics on children orphaned by AIDS in 88 countries, discusses the impact of AIDS on children, and discusses strategies for helping orphans and other children affected by AIDS.
Africa
Orphans and other children affected by HIV/AIDS. 3p col fig col map 2002 UNICEF, Programme Publs., 12-G, 3 UN Plaza, New York, NY 10017 single copy free; order or download at

Figure 4.12   Sample page from *Vertical File Index*

allow you to retrieve specifically that type of information. If, for example, you have already done a lot of research and don't need any of the articles written by John Doe, you may exclude them from your search. Or you (the searcher) may program the computer to advise you each month if anything new is published in your area of interest. (This service is called SDI—Selective Dissemination of Information.)

Some of the databases of specific interest to the researcher of nursing and health sciences that are now available online are:

- *Biotechnology Abstracts*
- *Chemline*
- *Clinical Abstracts*
- *Combined Health Information Database (CHID)*
- *Current Biotechnology Abstracts*
- *Diogenes*
- *Drug Information Fulltext*
- *Embase*
- *Information Online*
- *International Pharmaceutical Abstracts*
- *Life Sciences Collection*
- *Martindale Online*
- *Medline*
- *Mental Health Abstracts*
- *The Merck Index Online*
- *Nursing and Allied Health Index (CINAHL)*
- *Occupation Safety and Health (NIOSH)*
- *Pharmaceutical News Index*
- *Psychological Abstracts*
- *Sedbase*
- *Smoking and Health*
- *Toxnet*
- *Zoological Record*

Many of the other hundreds of available databases may also contain articles of interest to the nursing student, nurse, or health practitioner. Online searching is an extremely useful tool for the professional researcher. Everyone should at least be introduced to it.

Those who learn early in their career to use periodical indexes and to use them well will find that it makes their research easier and gives it a timeliness lacking in that of many of their colleagues.

Chapter Five

Electronic Resources and the Internet

"...The Good, the Bad, and the Ugly..."

The very first issue that must be dealt with in facing the world of electronic information is the issue of finding the *best* of all possible sources. Some researchers, particularly younger ones, exhibit a strong tendency to want to find everything in electronic format. Other users are especially resistant to anything that is not printed on paper. Good research lies at neither of those two extremes. What the excellent researcher *must* find is the *best* source of information to meet his or her needs, regardless of the format.

Depending on the nature of the query, both types of sources may be roughly equal or one may be far superior to the other. For example, a researcher already in the library needing to know the population of the world may find it much more quickly by approaching the reference librarian and asking the straightforward question, "What is the current world population?" In all likelihood, the reference librarian will quickly grab the latest edition of *World Almanac* from a shelf within arm's reach and have the figure in less than a minute—far faster than poking around on the World Wide Web, trying to locate a site that *might* have the information and then locating the information itself. Even from home or the office, the researcher might find it quicker to call the telephone reference service at the library and ask the question than to try to find it online.

On the other hand, if he needs the latest, most up-to-the-minute information, it is far more likely to be current in an online source such as the world population clock at http://www.biblio.org/lunarbin/worldpop or http://www.census.gov/cgi-bin/ipc/popclockw than in a print publication. It may be much better to use the online information even if it takes a while to determine that such a site exists and to discover its location.

Format has no bearing on the quality of information. No source is inherently better than another because of its format—though one may be easier to use, more current or more precise in locating the desired information than the other because of the usability its format provides. If the scholar is unsure whether a print or an online source would be the better choice, ask the person trained in locating and evaluating reference sources—the reference librarian.

Today's highly connected world is replete with electronic resources of all kinds. All these resources can be categorized into one of only two kinds: good ones and bad ones. Electronic resources need to be evaluated against the same criteria discussed in Chapter 3 under "Evaluating a Reference Book."

One of the main problems—and benefits—of the World Wide Web is that virtually anyone can mount Web pages and become an information provider. There is no control over who mounts the information, and no editing to keep the information correct and well-written.

Just as with a print source, the student should always ask:

- Who is the author of this information?

- Is he a reliable source?

- Is he an authority in the field?

- Who is the publisher? The fact that the information is mounted on a university server somewhere does not necessarily make it reliable; it could be information mounted on the Web page of a freshman student. Is the information endorsed by the university?

- What is the purpose of this information? Did the author mount the information as part of his scholarly research? Or was it mounted as part of his job? Did he mount the information in order to convince the world of his own point of view on a topic, regardless of the facts?

- Is the information current? When was it created or last updated? When is it likely to change again?

- In those cases where currency is important, how old is the information?

- Does the author show bias toward or against the subject? In today's world, it is all too common for individuals to mount an attack against another person or company. This attack may be open or sometimes hidden under the guise of "scholarly information."

- Is the information copyrighted? Original works of scholarship are considered property of their author and are protected under copyright law regardless of whether they bear notice of copyright or not—unless the author has explicitly stated that the work has been placed in the public domain. Even so, the scholar must make sure that the person saying he has placed the work in the public domain is its sole owner and entitled to do so. With electronic resources, it is far too easy to cut and paste information into a research paper without proper citation or acknowledgment of copyright.

- Is the work indexed? Perhaps an index is not quite so important in an electronic work as in a paper one because the scholar can often use a "find" or "search" function to locate the needed information. But the information needs to be well enough organized to be useful without wasting a lot of the researcher's time.

- How is the material organized? It is just as important for material to be logically organized in an electronic resource as in a print one, even though the limitation of poor organization may be easier to overcome in an electronic environment.

One of the major problems with electronic resources, particularly those mounted on the Internet and the World Wide Web, is that they may disappear quickly. It seems to be fairly common, for example, for a given university to maintain a Web site on a certain topic with reliable scholarly, authoritative information for several years. Then, the student who was maintaining the site graduates or the professor gets a new job, and the information ceases to be updated or disappears altogether.

Good Sources of Information

The serious researcher quickly discovers that the Internet is full of unreliable sources of questionable information. Are there any good sources out there? If so, what are some of them?

The Internet was created by the U.S. government for military purposes. It was quickly embraced by the academic and scholarly community as a way for researchers to share information quickly and efficiently. Only in the late 1990s, after the creation of the World Wide Web and as online tools became easier to use did the Internet begin to be dominated by the commercial sector. The government and scholarly sources of information haven't disappeared; they've just become harder to find in a very crowded world.

Always note the domain name of a site: ".com" usually indicates a commercial site; ".org" an organization, often not-for-profit; ".net" indicates a network of some type; and ".edu" is a U.S. institution of higher education. Two other domain types are ".gov" for sites belonging to the U.S. federal government and ".mil" for the U.S. military. The domain name can be a big clue as to the purpose of a Web site and a key to the type of information you can expect to find there.

It should be noted that the presence of a tilde character ("~") in the URL may be a significant clue to the validity of a Web site. The presence of a tilde in an address such as "http:// www.harvard.edu/~jones" may indicate that the page is maintained by a student or a faculty member named "Jones." In other words, the presence of ".edu" in a URL does not automatically indicate that the pages being viewed are authorized and/or maintained by the university.

Colleges and Universities

One of the best sources of information for the researcher is the college or university that conducts research in or specializes in a given discipline. Just as we might expect, you would not be disappointed by looking to the University of Maryland School of Nursing, http://nursing.umaryland.edu, or the Columbia University Nursing School, http://www.nursing.hs.columbia.edu for information in the area of nursing.

Colleges and universities that teach a particular discipline have often created Web sites with links to many useful resources in that discipline for their students. These sites are generally open to nonstudents as well. Thus, if you know that a school offers degrees in a certain field, you can look there as a starting point to find related resources rather than blindly searching the Web.

Obviously, many colleges and universities will offer majors in subject areas of interest to the student and scholar in nursing and allied health. Many of these sites provide excellent research materials, as well as links to other useful resources.

Government Resources

Governments gather data and create information. Because it's paid for with tax dollars, much of this information is in the public domain. Governments at all levels (city, state, federal, etc.) in many countries are now realizing that it may be less expensive for them to provide this information over the Internet than to produce multiple copies of large documents in a print version. This has created a pool of great wealth for the researcher.

The first step in using government information is for the researcher to determine which government body might have produced the information he needs. Which country would have produced the information? At what level would the information have been produced? At the federal level? The state or province level? The county or municipal level?

The next step is to determine *where* the information might have been produced. In the U.S., for example, information about a given state is likely to have been produced by that state, not by a state on the other side of the continent.

If the researcher is not sure where to begin a search, he should bear in mind that many governments have linked their sites to other government sites. For example, the U.S. federal government has established the National Contact Center at the Federal Citizen Information Center Internet site at http://fic.info.gov. The researcher can locate information on these sites by browsing or by using a search engine on the site to find information by keyword. At the FIC site, the researcher can find links to myriad federal government Web sites, as well as links to state and local government sites. Web sites are listed both by state and by topical subject area. In addition, some government bodies provide telephone numbers, sometimes toll-free, that the researcher can call for assistance in locating information.

Another useful site maintained by the U.S. federal government is FedWorld at http://www.fedworld.gov. FedWorld offers a gateway to many other government information systems as well as U.S. government reports and access to many other federal government Web sites.

The U.S. Government Printing Office, http://www.gpoaccess.gov, provides information on many topics, particularly those related to the federal government and legal matters.

Both houses of the U.S. Congress maintain Web sites at http://www.senate.gov and http://www.house.gov, respectively.

Two other important and useful federal government sites are the White House at http://www.whitehouse.gov and Thomas, a government information site maintained by the Library of Congress, at http://thomas.loc.gov.

Almost all state governments in the U.S. can be located with the Web address http://www.state.[postal abbreviation].us; for example, http://www.state.ca.us for California or http://www.state.tx.us for Texas. The abbreviation used for the state is the official postal code used by the U.S. Postal Service. On their sites, states have links to county and city government sites. Many states also provide links to the federal government and to other states.

There are links to all United Kingdom government authorities at the CCTA Government Information Service Web site at http://www.open.gov.uk.

Entire books have been written about U.S. and other government Internet sites. The researcher expecting to need to use such information is well advised to acquire some of these.

Organizations

As the World Wide Web has grown in popularity, virtually every not-for-profit organization of any size has established a Web site. These sites provide much information freely available to all. Because of the nature of these organizations, such information is generally ample and authoritative. Examples of such groups would be the American Cancer Society at http://www.cancer.org or the American Heart Association, http://www.americanheart.org.

Hobbyists, collectors, and aficionados of all types have created Web sites around their mutual interest. Such sites include the American Numismatic Association at http://www.money.org or Collectors.Org at http://www.collectors.org. Two examples of personal nurse's Web sites are Pam's Place on the Web, http://www.cp-tel.net/pam north, and Jenny's Homepage at http://www.geocities.com/jen2y1973. Pam is an RN working in hospice care in Louisiana; Jenny is a Filipino nurse working in the U.S.

Many nursing organizations and societies have their own Web sites. Often these sites can provide valuable links to other resources. Some examples include the American Nurses Association at http://www.nursingworld.org, the National League for Nursing at http://www.nln.org, and HealthWeb at http://healthweb.org.

Many professional societies now have information available online to members and nonmembers alike, such as the American Medical Association, http://www.ama-assn. org, or the American Psychological Association at http://www.apa.org. The American Nurses Association (ANA) has a Web site at http://www.ana.org. The Association of PeriOperative Registered Nurses (AORN) has a site at http://www. aorn.org.

Libraries

Librarians are specialists in organizing information. Just as they have organized books and materials within the library for many years, many librarians are now organizing information outside the library walls by establishing Web sites with many resources useful to the researcher, particularly links to other useful sites.

The primary starting place for a researcher in the U.S. might well be the Library of Congress at http://www.loc.gov, while the researcher in Britain might want to start with The British Library at http://portico.bl.uk. The National Library of Canada can be located at http://www.nlc-bnc.ca. Similarly, many other countries have their own national libraries, which have links to other libraries, including libraries in other countries, as well as state or provincial and local libraries.

In the U.S., most states have an official state library or library agency. Unfortunately, the address pattern varies from state to state, so while the State Library of Indiana can be found at http://www.statelib.lib.in.us, the address for the State Library of California is not www.statelib.lib.ca.us. A list of links to state libraries and agencies can be found at http://www.dpi.state.wi.us/dpi/dlcl/pld/statelib.html. There is also a list at http://sunsite.berkeley.edu/Libweb/usa-state.html.

Some library networks are combining their efforts to provide a suite of online databases freely available to all the residents of their particular state. A few prime examples are SAILOR, Maryland's Online Public Information Network, http://www.sailor.lib.md.us; ACLIN, Colorado Virtual Library, http://www.aclin.org; Galileo, Georgia Library Learning Online, http://www.galileo.usg.edu; and INSPIRE, Indiana Spectrum of Information Resources, http://www.inspire.net.

An increasing number of libraries are offering online reference services, not only to their particular constituents, but to anyone. If the researcher can wait from 24 to 48 hours for a response to a query, this may be an excellent source of information. The user enters the query online via the library's Web page and receives the answer by e-mail. One such site is the Internet Public Library at http://www.ipl.org.

Some libraries are specialists in specific-subject areas, so visiting one of those sites can lead the researcher to many other useful sites on that particular topic. Ask the reference librarian for information on good sites for specific topics.

Commercial Enterprises

Although the Internet was originally dominated by government, education, and military sectors, today one of the largest types of suppliers of information via the Internet is the commercial sector. Many of these companies offer goods and services for sale, while others offer information and wares at no charge in exchange for wading through the commercial advertisements that sponsor the site. Certainly, the scholar in nursing and health sciences will find sites such as bookstores and publishers useful.

Among the better-known bookstores on the Web are Amazon.com at http://www.amazon.com and Barnes and Noble at http://www.barnesandnoble.com.

In addition to bookstores and publishers, almost every type of business imaginable has a presence on the World Wide Web. Without knowing the exact address of the company, it is often possible to locate the company simply by guessing that the address is probably www.company-name.com. Many of these sites are authorities in their field, offering the user much helpful information and often leading to other useful sites.

Electronic Journals

There are thousands of journals and magazines available via the World Wide Web. Like their print counterparts, these range from scholarly to general interest to limited interest. In fact, some of them seem to come and go so quickly that they are probably in a class called "no interest."

Also, like their print counterparts, these electronic journals run the gamut from excellent to poor. At the top end are the scholarly journals. In some cases, these journals are exact versions of their print equivalent, while others are limited, providing only a table of contents or a few select articles.

At the bottom of the ladder are the "Ezines," magazines often published for a relatively limited special-interest group. Depending on the topic and the writers, these can range from excellent to worthless and must be read while applying the same measurements for quality reference sources previously outlined.

Some of these publications, particularly the scholarly journals, may be available only via subscription, and often at a high price. A good first stop is the library, which may have purchased a subscription for its patrons.

Other sites are highly commercial and freely available to the reader and are supported by the online ads you must view in order to read the publication. Some may be free to the user and free of commercial affiliations, perhaps because they are published by a scholarly society by and for its members, or because someone publishes them as a labor of love to support a particular interest. Quality varies widely. As may be expected, some are excellent and some are not worth the electrons they're written with.

Electronic publications may be valuable sources of information, but in today's world, they have not yet achieved the scholarly acceptance of print resources, unless they are the electronic version of the same title in print.

Online News Media

Every type of journalism medium that we are familiar with has now migrated to the World Wide Web: magazines, newspapers, radio stations, and TV stations. Any medium that didn't want to be left behind has now made the journey. Often, the sources we are already familiar with can be good sources for instant information. Need to check the weather but it's not time for the local news? Check the Web site of the local TV station. Do you know of a story that was featured in yesterday's newspaper but you didn't get to buy a copy? Check the newspaper's Web site. There is a list of newspapers, organized by location or subject at NewsDirectory.com, http://news-directory.com. Want to know what time a particular show will be on television this evening? Check the Web site of the local TV station, newspaper, or perhaps even the affiliated radio station. BRS Web-Radio provides a directory of U.S. radio stations searchable by call letters, state, or format at http://www.web-radio.com. It also includes international and Internet-only stations. TV Station Web Page Directory offers a directory of television station Web sites searchable by location at http://www3. sympatico.ca/ralway/tvdirect/welcome.html.

Search Engines

In the early to mid-1990s before the Internet became more commercial and moved into the public domain, there was a lot of information available from government and academic sources, but it was practically impossible to find. About the only way to find information back then was to know its location—which the researcher often did not.

As much of the Internet migrated to the World Wide Web in the mid- to late-1990s, we saw the development of the search engine. These services, usually paid for by commercial advertising, and therefore free to the end-user, routinely search and index many of the sites on the Internet. Basically, these services can be divided into four categories.

1. General Search Engines

General search engines, as the name describes, index sites and information of all types, regardless of subject or location or language.

There are numerous general search engines available on the Web, with the number changing almost daily as new search engines appear and others merge with or are bought out by the competition. A few of the general search engines are listed in the appendix, but the researcher must bear in mind that the name and address of these resources may have changed or disappeared before this book sees print.

There are several important factors the researcher must remember about these search engines:

- Search engines run a program—often called a crawler, robot, worm, or some other name—which searches the Internet daily, often a different part of the Net each day, until completing its rotation and beginning again. The information these programs retrieve is placed into a database and indexed. When the user searches the Web using one of these search engines, he is really searching just the database created by the robot, which has already searched the Web and retrieved some information. Because the Net is searched in segments, the information in the database may not be the most up-to-date; it is simply what the crawler found the day it searched.

- The search engines retrieve and index whatever they find; no attempt is made to evaluate the quality of the sites or to differentiate between sites that are definitive and those containing erroneous or false information.

- Not all search engines will return the same results for an identical search. There are several reasons for this:

  - Search engines do not find and index the same sites. In fact, a 1998 study determined that no single search engine indexed even as much as 50 percent of the estimated 320 million Web pages available.[1]

  - Each search engine uses its own criteria to assign index terms to the data it has placed into its database. Because the indexing is automated, it may or may not be accurate.

  - When a user performs a search for information, each search engine uses its own set of algorithms to determine the relevance of a Web document to the search terms.[2] The algorithms are based on such factors as how many times the sought-after term occurs; whether the term occurs in the title of the document, a header, or within the text; the proximity of one search term to another within the document; the number of terms from the document that match the query; and numerous other factors. Not all search engines use the same factors. In any case, each search engine places a different value on each of these factors.

With all these variables, it is easy to see why different search engines may return different sets of documents:

- Because the request for information is interpreted and analyzed by computer software with no human intervention, the search results can be only as good as an engine's retrieval algorithm. A poorly written formula will either miss important documents or return many irrelevant ones—or both.

- Not all search engines allow the same search options. For example, one search engine may allow a search to be restricted by date or language, whereas another may not, thereby leading to different results.

Finally, the researcher needs to learn something about proper searching techniques. The proper way to conduct a search is not to go to one of the general search engines and directly type in the question, such as "What are the best practices for nursing care of a stroke patient?" as novice searchers often do. Rather, the searcher should use the general search engine to locate Web sites dealing with the topic, in this case "stroke," then search those stroke-related Web sites for the desired information.

The best advice for the researcher seeking breadth and depth of information is to use more than one search engine to locate the desired information.

2. Specialized Search Engines

Another type of search engine is the specialized search engine. These search engines can be categorized by the subject matter they cover or by the type of sites they index. Usually these search engines are limited to a specific format or subject area:

- **http://groups.google.com** Google Groups is an index to the messages posted in Usenet discussion forums.
- **http://healthcentral.com** Healthcentral provides consumer health information and news about health products.
- **http://www.hon.ch** Health on the Net Foundation, a nongovernmental organization whose mission is to guide laypeople and others to useful and reliable online medical information.
- **http://www.mednets.com** A medical search engine and health portal.

Whereas the general search engine attempts to search any information that is available on the World Wide Web, the specialized search engine attempts only to locate and index resources of a given type or in a certain subject area. The result is that a specialized search engine *may* yield information that is more relevant to the topic and easier for the searcher to find without retrieving a lot of irrelevant information. If the researcher can locate a search engine in his area of interest, it can be a much better source to use than a general search engine.

3. Metasearch Engines

The difference between a metasearch engine and the general search engine is that a metasearch engine allows the user to enter the search terms once and search multiple search engines simultaneously. There are, however, a couple of important cautions in using metasearch engines:

- Some metasearch engines limit the number of documents retrieved from each search engine, often to between 10 and 25 items.

- The program may time-out before the search engine has had time to retrieve all the relevant documents.

- The search terms entered into the metasearch engine may not be treated the same way by each search engine. For example, terms may have been entered using a Boolean "and" in the metasearch engine but the "and" is ignored by the general search engine and the terms are "or"ed together, resulting in a great number of irrelevant documents.

In conclusion, a metasearch engine may be a good starting place or a great time-saver in a pinch, but the researcher who wants great breadth and depth of information should not rely on a metasearch engine alone.

4. Directories

Directories should not be confused with search engines, though some sites, such as Yahoo!, have search capabilities as well as a directory. A directory is a site that has information arranged into hierarchical categories by subject, such as "education," "science," "social sciences," "entertainment," "travel," "news," and "weather."

Because these categories have been organized with human intervention—sometimes by librarians or information specialists—they may be quicker and easier to search and yield more precise results than a general search engine. For example, a search for "travel" on AltaVista, http://www.altavista.com, yielded 29,574,298 results; a search for "'travel' and 'Oxford'" yielded 2,089,810 Web pages.[3] A search through the AltaVista directories allowed us to go from the top level through "Travel & Vacations," "Europe," "Great Britain," "Regional England," "Central & Eastern," to various travel guides on Oxford, our destination, in only five mouse clicks.

Of course, some topics, such as "travel" and "entertainment," are popular and easy to find in the directories, whereas other topics, particularly those of more limited interest, may be impossible, or nearly so, to find through the directories, sometimes because of too many hits. A search for "experience based practice" on Google, for example yielded 26 hits, whereas a search for "pressure sores" resulted in 29,600 items.

Many of the problems with using search engines were well summarized by Randolph Hock:

> Unfortunately—and the impact of this continues into the present—none of the search engines took advantage of the heavy-duty searching technology and approaches found in online services such as Dialog and LexisNexis. Neither did the search engines nor their cousins, the Web directories, take advantage of the extensive subject classification theory and practice of the last hundred or so years.[4]

An increasing number of the general search engines are developing a directory structure in addition to their search engine. The researcher seeking such a structure might well start by visiting the page of one of these search engines.

Much valuable background and current information about search engines can be found at Search Engine Watch, http://www.searchenginewatch.com.

Online Search Services

Online search services, like Dialog and LexisNexis, have been around for many years and, through libraries, have been available to the general public longer than the Internet and the World Wide Web. Dialog Corporation, for example, became the world's first commercial online service in 1972.

How do these online services differ from what's generally available over the Internet? First of all, these services are not free. Many of these services require a subscription for a searcher to access their services, thus requiring that the researcher know in advance that he is going to use the services. As some of these services are quite expensive, the occasional searcher will want to access them through his employer or through the library. Many public, academic, and corporate libraries are subscribers to these online services.

Charges are calculated on a number of factors:

- *Subscription charge.* Sometimes there is a subscription charge just to access the service. Sometimes some or all of this charge may be considered a prepay and is credited against future use of the services. If the user is accessing the service through a library or some other entity, that organization will be the one to pay the subscription fee.

- *Telecommunications charges.* The user must pay a telecommunication charge to connect to the online service. If the access is available via the Internet, there may be no telecommunications charge or only a modest one from the vendor to offset the expense of making that type of connection available. If the user must access the service directly, this charge may appear in the form of a long-distance phone call from the user's location to the location of the provider's computer.

- *Connection charges.* Sometimes there is a connection charge for accessing a particular database. Even if there is no activity, the user may be charged for the amount of time he is connected to the database. Therefore, it is advisable that the user be prepared to conduct the search quickly and get offline to analyze the results. As some databases are less expensive than others, the user may want to create the search in a cheaper database, save it, and then transfer it to the more expensive database. Connection charges can range all the way from a few dollars per hour to hundreds of dollars per hour.

- *Activity charges.* Some search services may levy activity charges instead of or in addition to connection charges. Activity charges are based on the database being searched and the amount of processor time used by the computer in conducting the search. A more difficult search will take more computer time and, therefore, be more expensive. Likewise, a search retrieving many items may take longer and be more expensive than one that retrieves few items.

- *Citation charges.* Users may be charged for each citation retrieved. The amount charged will vary with the type of information viewed; for example, citations only, citations with abstracts, or full text. Obviously, full text will be the more expensive option.

- *Print charges.* There may be a print charge for some citations. Again, the charges will vary depending on the format requested. Charges will also vary depending on the retrieval method: whether viewed online, sent via e-mail, faxed, or printed offline and sent via regular mail.

- *Local service charges.* Some organizations, such as the library, may levy a service charge to pay for maintaining the equipment, the connection, and the time and training of the person who conducts the search for the user.

Naturally, the more quickly and accurately a search can be performed, the lower the cost. The logical conclusion is that it's often most cost-effective to have a librarian or professional searcher conduct the search for the researcher.

The databases available through these services have been created and maintained by librarians and subject experts in their particular area. Therefore, the articles contained therein are most likely to be of interest to the professional researcher and may have been screened for quality and accuracy.

Web pages are generally not created to be searchable but to be viewed. Because these databases are created to be searchable and are created by professionals, the information is usually divided into fields and subfields for greater precision in information retrieval. Their search engines are specially created to take advantage of these search handles. The end result is that the retrieval of records can be more precise and quicker.

Local Databases

Many libraries may own or subscribe to databases either on a local server or on CD-ROM. Many of these databases are those that the researcher would have to pay to use if trying to access them directly or over the Internet. These databases may be accessible over the library's network or, if on CD-ROM, they may be available for checkout—both in-house and external—from the library's circulation or reference desk. Some of them may be available to the library patron from home via dialup or the Internet. Ask which ones your library has that may be of interest to you and how you can get access.

Some of these databases may be of highly local interest and available nowhere else. Some examples would be an index to the local newspaper, or at least its obituaries; a database of flowers or birds of the state or region.

Libraries and Internet Access

As we've already mentioned, many libraries now have Internet access. This benefits the researcher in numerous ways.

First of all, if the user does not have Internet access from home or the office, it's often available through the local public or university library. The resources of a library are no longer limited to those contained within its walls.

Because libraries specialize in providing information, they may likely have had other patrons performing research in your major subject area. The reference staff may know of useful Internet resources to which they can point you.

In addition, the library may have created "pathfinders" or bibliographies in various subject areas. These may be in print form containing a list of Internet sites relevant to that topic, or they may be online, permitting the user direct access to the resources via the hyperlinks contained in the document.[5]

Other Online Databases

The library or educational institution may provide its users or students with access to other databases and resources that the user would normally have to pay a subscription fee to access. The difference between these databases and those mentioned previously under "online Search Services" is that most of these charge a flat fee rather than a per-use fee. Thus, the institution pays a specific amount for access to the resource—usually an annual fee—and users can access it as much as they want with no additional charges incurring to them or to the library.

Many of these databases are from commercial concerns such as H.W. Wilson or EBSCO. In some cases, they may be provided to the library by state and local or regional consortia. Some of the databases may have been created by the library.

Document Delivery

The purpose of a document delivery service is, as the name says, to provide documents for the researcher. In most cases, we are referring to documents that are less than book length, as book-length manuscripts can be obtained using the interlibrary loan services of the researcher's library.

The suppliers are companies or organizations, often commercial, which can retrieve almost anything for a fee. A quick-and-dirty definition might be, "we can get almost anything you can pay for" though this hardly does justice to the many libraries and not-for-profit organizations that provide this service for the benefit of the researcher, seeking only to cover their costs.

A researcher may find a reference to a specific document either through his reading, on the Web, or through online searching. It may be that the desired document, such as an article in a copyrighted journal, is not freely available in electronic form. Or, perhaps the researcher is not near a library where the document might be retrieved. This is the gap that a document delivery service is meant to fill.

Some document delivery services may contain search engines or subject indexes that the researcher can use to locate relevant articles. Others may not. Regardless of how the citation is discovered, it is the function of the document delivery service to produce the article for the user.

First, let us clarify a couple of points: A document delivery service does not usually provide original documents. A document delivery service would not be the place to request an original folio of Shakespeare. It may, however, be able to provide a photocopy or electronic facsimile of that folio. Essentially, document delivery services are able to provide documents that can be photocopied or scanned into electronic format, or that are already available in electronic format.

As the first step in retrieving a document, the researcher must locate an accurate citation. If the citation information is inaccurate, it is quite likely that the retrieval service will be unable to locate the document.

Next, the researcher contacts the document delivery service. These days that generally means via the World Wide Web, but it could be via fax, a phone call, or even via regular mail.

After receiving the request, the retrieval service will inform the researcher whether or not it is able to provide the requested document, at what cost, in what form, and within what time period. If the researcher is accessing the service via the Web, this information may be returned immediately.

It must here be noted that document delivery services are generally commercial concerns that charge for their services. Some require a prepaid subscription for the user even to be able to access their services.

While some services may not require a prepaid subscription, such a subscription may allow the user to retrieve documents at a discount from the price paid by the general public. A researcher should inquire at his or her local library if such an arrangement exists.

Other services require no such prepaid arrangement but are able to provide documents on-demand to the individual user. Such an arrangement is useful to the occasional user who may request only one or two documents at a time. Payment is generally made online via a credit card. Many of the services provide secure sites for the sending of such sensitive information. It must be noted, however, that transactions in some countries or transactions between countries may not be totally secure. Some services will allow a user to enter all the citation information directly via the Web, while they provide a phone number (sometimes toll-free) for the user who does not want to provide credit card information online.

The cost of a document may vary and is comprised of the copyright fee that the user must pay in order to use this document, plus what the retrieval service charges for its services, and sometimes a copying fee based on the number of pages. The fee per document may vary depending on several factors including the length of the document, the amount of the copyright fee, and the method of delivery. Two different delivery services may charge vastly different prices for the same document.

While requesting the document, the user will indicate a preferred method of delivery. Some documents that exist in electronic format may be accessed directly online once the fee is paid and may sometimes be printed directly if desired. Or, documents may be sent via regular mail, e-mail, or fax. If the requested document exists only in paper format, the fee sometimes pays for converting that document to electronic format so that the user can access it directly over the Web after it has been converted.

The document delivery market is currently undergoing major transition, and the user is cautioned to do diligent research into which may be the best service to use. Bear in mind, of course, that it may be desirable to use more than a single source from time to time.

A list of document delivery providers is given in the appendix, with the caution that things are changing rapidly in this field and any company listed may have been sold or dismantled after press time.

Current Awareness Services

There are services that scholars can use to maintain constant awareness of what's being newly published in their field or areas of interest. These services, often called "current awareness services" or "selective dissemination of information (SDI)," periodically provide to the researcher a report on what's been newly published on specific topics. Most of these services function in the following manner:

> The scholar locates a supplier, tells the supplier what his areas of interest are, how often he needs to receive the information (daily, weekly, etc.), and how much information he needs to receive (table of contents, article citations, abstracts, etc.), and contracts with the supplier. The price for the service may be based on some combination of the frequency of updates, the type of information supplied, and the amount of information supplied.

While this can be an expensive option, it is an excellent way for the researcher to stay at the forefront of his field.

Untested Resources

There are literally hundreds of millions of documents and information sources available via the Internet and the World Wide Web. Availability does not equate with quality. Many of the sources are created by people with little knowledge of their topic or with a particular vendetta or axe to grind. Some of this information is provided by undergraduate students who are just beginning to study in their fields, or even by high school students and younger—often without any indication of who the author is or what his particular level of expertise is in this topic area. Check to determine the date of the information provided; accurate information is often rendered useless by the passage of time. And if possible, try to ascertain whether the information will be available into the future; as noted previously, resources produced by students or by a particular class often disappear or become static when those students move on.

The diligent researcher will examine his sources carefully (whether electronic or otherwise) and apply to them the same criteria used in determining the validity of any reference source.

Free Databases

Some individuals or organizations have mounted databases on the Web, which are searchable by anyone at no charge. Some of these databases are limited by subject type:

- The PubMed Database, http://www.ncbi.nlm.nih.gov/entrez/query.fcgi, is searchable by subject, keywords, authors, title, or journal name.
- Health-e-Links, http://www.healthelinks.org, directs you to other health sources.
- The Rehab Database, http://www.naric.com/search/rhab, is a database on disability and rehabilitation, searchable by author, title, and descriptor.

As always, examine the source in order to evaluate the validity of the information.

Electronic Mailing Lists and Discussion Groups

Mailing lists and discussion groups are like the town square of the Internet: Anyone with an idea, opinion, advice, thought, etc., is allowed to voice it. Anyone else is allowed to agree or disagree. There are lists and groups on every topic imaginable and some that most of us would never imagine!

The interested person locates a discussion group, mailing list, or newsgroup of interest and then electronically subscribes. Mailing lists and newsgroups are technologically slightly different, the main difference being that with a mailing list, a copy of every post lands in the subscriber's mailbox and stays there until it is deleted, while newsgroup postings are available for a time and then disappear whether you act on them or not. Some newsgroups may simply be viewed without actually subscribing.

Whenever someone has a question or something to share, he sends a message to the address of the group. Everyone in the group receives a copy of that message. All responses (except those that are purposely directed to an individual) go to the entire group. The group member can either participate in the discussion or simply view it (called "lurking").

A list of lists and newsletters can be found at http://www.liszt.com. Topica, formerly Liszt, is a search engine where you can search for discussion groups or newsletters on the topic(s) of choice. A search for "nursing" yielded four categories. A search for lists dealing with "health & fitness" turned up 12 categories.

The information given about each list includes:

- The list name

- The name of the computer that hosts the list

- The name of the contact person(s)

- A description of the list

- Where to get more info

- How to subscribe and unsubscribe

- A few newsgroups of possible interest to the researcher in nursing and health sciences:

  - Nursingnetwork, http://www.nursingnetwork.com

  - Critical Care Nursing List (CCN-L), http://www.icustat.com

  - The No Fluff Zone newsletter, http://www.nurseserver.com

  - NSG Informatics, Informatics-subscribe@topica.com

The archives of many discussion groups formerly at http://www.deja.com, can now be found on google.groups.com. Because newsgroups are resource-intensive, requiring vast amounts of storage space, and because some are quite controversial,[6] not all newsgroups are carried by every Internet provider. "Although most newsgroups cater to aboveboard hobbies, there's a share of pornographic, incendiary, provocative, and plain moronic material."[7] Some providers may carry all groups, some may carry only select groups, and others may carry none at all. The researcher should ask his provider if access to newsgroups is available and how.

Webrings

Webrings are in a category that falls somewhere between the reliable and the untested sources, as there may be Webrings of both types. A Webring is merely a consortium of independently mounted sites with pointers to each other. The ring may simply come into existence spontaneously as people with a common interest share resources, may be semi-organized as participants request that each site comply with specific guidelines, or be formally organized with adherence to specific behaviors being part of the price of joining. The latter may be monitored for reliability and conformity. Unfortunately, the scholar often has nothing other than the word of the sites themselves to vouch for their validity.

In a Webring, each site may point to all other sites or they may be organized rotationally—that is, site one points to site two, site two points to site three, etc., with the last site pointing back to the first (i.e., in a ringlike fashion).

Because Webrings are often mounted by hobbyists, scholars, or those with a particular common interest, they are good places to locate information that is not found elsewhere because it is too esoteric or of limited interest. Because of the interest of the participants in their topic, these sites may provide a depth and breadth of information not available elsewhere. The scholar needs to investigate judiciously the source of the information and determine its reliability before depending on it.

Webrings can provide pointers to Web sites, particularly smaller ones, which may not have been indexed by the major search engines.

If the search terms you would use to locate a specific topic are too generic or have multiple meanings, a Webring may be the best starting place for locating other similar sites. The key is locating the first site in the ring—an often difficult task. The best starting place may be one of the general search engines or a college or university site offering studies in that particular subject area.

A good starting point is WebRing, variously listed as http://www.webring.com, http://www.webring.org, and http://www.webring.net (all roads lead to Rome). WebRing lists several dozen rings related to nursing. A less well-organized site but interesting for browsing is The Rail at http://www.therail.com.

Community Networks

Community networks are another category that falls between reliable and untested resources, depending on the source of the information contained. A single network may contain information running the gamut from very reliable to totally discreditable.

"Community" bears a variety of definitions, ranging from one city or town only to countywide or regionwide. These networks are electronic networks, usually consisting of a series of Web pages pointing to various resources of information on the local community. Such resources might include information on the area, its businesses, libraries, and community groups, and other resources such as chat rooms or mailing lists. As might be expected, much of the information is of great local interest or of interest to someone studying that particular area.

If you know where a resource (such as a college or university library) is located geographically but do not know its Web address, you might be able to locate the electronic resource via the network of the community where the institution is located.

One of the first community networks in the United States was the Michiana Free-Net, http://michiana.org. Other well-known examples are Chicago Mosaic, http://www.ci.chi.il.us; San Diego Source, http://www.sddt.com; and Austin Free-Net, http://www.austinfree.net.

Citing Electronic Resources

Because electronic resources are in a different format than print resources and because they tend to appear and disappear quickly, they require a different form of bibliographic entry. Some of the standard bibliographic guides, such as the *MLA Style Guide*, now devote a section to or have a separate guide on citing electronic resources, and some new guides specifically for citing electronic information have appeared. Sample guides are listed in the bibliography.

Endnotes

1. Lawrence, S.R. and C. L. Giles. "Searching the World Wide Web" *Science* 280 (1998):98–100.

2. An algorithm is a set of criteria that a search engine uses to automatically analyze a document to determine whether it is appropriate to the information being requested.

3. As an example of how quickly things change, the exact same search was performed a few minutes later, resulting in 2,252,820 documents. A few weeks later, it yielded 2,415,580 Web pages.

4. Hock, Randolph. *The Extreme Searcher's Guide to Web Search Engines, Second Edition.* Medford, NJ: CyberAge Books, 2001.

5. "Hypertext" or "hyperlinks" are electronic links from the document currently being viewed by the reader to further information. Hyperlinks are usually readily visible within the text. The current convention is for a hyperlink to be blue and underlined, though this is not universally followed. By clicking on the link with the mouse, the user is transferred directly to the information being referred to. The user is cautioned that after connecting to a hyperlink, he may no longer be viewing a document created or maintained by the creator of the original document, and the information contained therein may or may not be reliable.

6. One well-known characteristic of newsgroups is that there is at least one group to offend everybody.

7. Kennedy, Angus J. *The Internet: The Rough Guide.* London: Rough Guides Ltd, 1998, p. 129.

Chapter Six

The Research Paper—
Putting It All Together

It has been said that the only *good* research paper is the *written* research paper. No matter how well the research has been executed or how many resources have been found and examined or how profound the insight into the subject as a result of a vigorous effort in the university library, it is to no avail until the research is written up in a coherent form.

This follow-through, the putting it all together, is addressed in this chapter. Our treatment will be brief; it will be simple but hopefully not simplistic. If the researcher needs more guidance than is offered here, it is available—from the professor, from the library staff, from well-written guides developed for that purpose. Substantial and detailed guides for paper writing may be purchased in the bookstores of most universities, and the better ones are also found in most libraries. But for our purposes here, what follows is what we think to be a sufficient guide for the researcher in the development of an above-average research paper or project.

Essentially, two procedures are necessary to bring a good paper to fruition; namely, a sound search strategy for the gathering of pertinent information, and then a well-developed organizational framework for the actual writing of the paper.

Search Strategy Model

The search strategy is a prerequisite to all research paper projects. The strategy, as illustrated in Figure 6.1, consists of three primary steps.

First, in order for a researcher to write a research paper she must develop a topic that derives from a subject area. Eventually, a well-thought-out topic will produce a descriptive title for the actual paper. For the student of nursing (or any student or researcher for that matter), an immediate perusal of the background sources constitutes the first step.

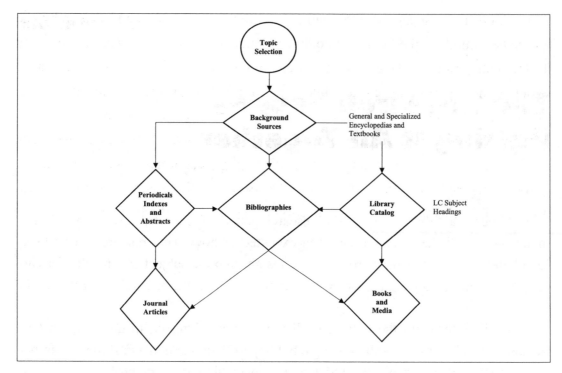

Figure 6.1   Search strategy model

The background sources are those general and specialized encyclopedias cited earlier—as well as the textbook if the research is being conducted for a course. (Students often fail to think of the required text in the course as a reference but it most certainly is.)

Another, and probably more effective and time-saving, method for the student of nursing and health sciences would be to go immediately to *Cumulative Index to Nursing and Allied Health Literature (CINAHL) Subject Index,* which is usually divided into two parts. Look at the subject headings in the volumes. There are hundreds of possibilities from which you may choose a topic for your research. Eventually there will be a subject that even the most unanimated researcher will find interesting. If you find a subject that is of particular interest to you, make a photocopy of that subject and the citations that appear beneath it. As you review these subject headings, note how many references there are under each of the headings. If there are many references, chances are that it will be easier for you to find more materials on that subject in the library that you are using. You can then use these citations to search for the original source materials in your library.

Look up an article and read through it. It will probably be short and written by one of the best minds in the field. If it holds your attention, then either make a photocopy of the bibliography at the end of the article, or copy the entire article making sure to write on the first page the entire bibliographical reference, namely, essay author, title of the article, volume, page numbers, and date and place of publication.

Now, having first consulted the background sources and identified a subject area (still far removed from the final topic and title of the research paper itself, but certainly a start in the right direction), proceed to the second level of research: the movement from the identification of a subject area to the development of a topic of research.

Topic Development

There are three components of this topic development area. The researcher will consult three very different, but related, areas of information identification.

First Step

First, consult the periodicals indexes and abstracts, and direct special interest and attention toward the *Cumulative Index to Nursing and Allied Health Literature* (*CINAHL*) (and book review indexes where applicable). In these sources, you should look up articles in each of several volumes (or online by keywords), usually beginning with the most recent volume and working backward until a substantial amount of literature has been identified. This will vary depending on the area and the topic being pursued, of course.

You should certainly identify a few articles in *CINAHL*, checking the periodicals holdings list to make sure that the articles that are included in the developing bibliography for the research paper are actually available in the library. (If they are not, and if there is sufficient time, you can always call for these articles through the interlibrary loan department or turn to a document delivery service). The subject area chosen while perusing *Mosby's Medical, Nursing, and Allied Health Dictionary* should be identified by one, two, or three words, called "keyword indicators." These words should be looked up in *CINAHL*. For example, such keywords might be "Patient Classification System," "Nursing Process," "Educational Levels," etc.

Second Step

The next step in the search strategy is to consult the *Bibliographic Index* and look up the keyword indicators to see if there is already a well-developed and reasonably recent bibliography on the subject area that you are interested in pursuing. If so, much of your work has already been done, for the development of an effective bibliography constitutes a major component in any research effort.

Finally, after gathering a few articles from *CINAHL* (making sure to get complete bibliographic information and not using any abbreviations but writing out every word completely to avoid possible confusion later on), go to the library catalog and look up the keywords for a listing of books and related materials held in the library stacks.

Before proceeding to the third step in this search strategy model, we feel compelled to say more about the notes being taken at this point. You are not yet taking notes on the research topic because it is not yet well developed. However, you should be armed with a stack of 3″ x 5″ or 4″ x 6″ cards, on which each bibliographic reference is written—one reference per card only. The complete bibliographic notation should include author, title, periodical, volume, issue number, date, pages, as well as the source of the reference, in this instance, *CINAHL*, and indicating which volume and page number. If you don't take down this information in its entirety, more than likely much time will be taken up in wasted steps retracing search procedures and countless hours spent redoing what should have been done in the first place.

It is a good idea to have a standard form on which to record the needed information. Figure 6.2 provides a suggested format for such a card. You may wish to duplicate a number of these cards ahead of time, and then, when a reference is found, just fill in the information, remembering to avoid abbreviations. If you work on a word processor, you can simply re-create the form in Figure 6.2 and copy it multiple times. Then you can decide whether it works best for you to print the forms on paper or cards or to fill in the form electronically. If you fill in the forms electronically, you can later print the documents and cut the forms apart to perform the sorting process described later.

This point about not abbreviating is being belabored here for a purpose. For example, if you locate in the *CINAHL* a reference to a splendid article in *AJN* and record the reference as such, by the time you get ready to locate the journal, you may have forgotten the exact and complete title of that specific reference. Then what? Probably a retracing of the reference by means of returning to the *CINAHL* and checking the reference index to find out that *AJN* is the *American Journal of Nursing*. If the full title had been recorded once and first, no retracing would need to be done—time saved.

Author(s)				
Title of Article				
Journal title				
Vol.	No.	Month	Year	Pages
Place of Publication, publisher, date, edition (books only)				
Library where info is located			Call #	
Source of Citation				
How item relates to research problem				
Use reverse side for additional comment. (If used, check here) ❏				

Figure 6.2   Bibligraphic note card

In the front of almost all reference indexes, in this instance *CINAHL*, there is a key to the abbreviations used in the body of the index, which you may refer to if in doubt about the correct and full title of certain periodicals. Remember that your note cards will later serve as the master bibliographic file when you are writing the actual paper. If you make them complete from the outset they will constitute a major help in subsequent writing.

Third Step

Step three in the search strategy model is actually using the sources of information, namely, the periodicals and the books identified in the preceding step. The books can usually be taken out of the library (unless they are categorized as rare books or reference works). The periodical literature often may not be. However, most libraries have copying facilities at minimal cost. Researchers are wise to copy the major articles to be used in their research, thus allowing them to move about with their research portfolio. Otherwise, the note-taking step must occur within the confines of the library, probably in the Bound Periodicals Room. Likewise, articles in electronic format should be printed or saved to disk.

The search has ended. The materials have been identified. This process, once rehearsed, can be executed in an hour or so. A researcher who has been trained in this system of library usage skills can enter the library without any notion of a topic and, in less than an hour, develop a respectable working bibliography.

At this juncture, you must begin to concentrate seriously upon the organizational model of the research. By now you have moved from no subject area to the discovery, thanks to the *Mosby's Medical, Nursing, and Allied Health Dictionary*, of a viable and interesting subject area.

Furthermore, you have developed the subject area—owing to the three-fold utilization of the search strategy model with *CINAHL*, the *Bibliographic Index,* and the library catalog—into an identifiable topic, and have a working bibliography to prove it. Now, you must become acquainted with the materials identified, gleaned, and collected appropriate to the topic.

Knowing and Owning the Materials

1. Quick Perusal

Quickly review all the materials you have gathered—two-dozen articles or so plus a particularly appropriate book or two on the topic. (Articles, not books, constitute the substance of library research in nursing and health sciences.) If you have photocopies of the articles, discreetly highlight and mark them at particularly important points. The idea here is a general acquaintance with the materials.

2. Outline Development

Develop an outline. Most research papers at this level will have three to five major components with three or four subheadings under each of those. Without an outline, the paper can hardly have a sense of developed logic and reasoned organization to it. The all-too-common practice of writing the outline after the paper has already been written is like drawing up architectural plans for a house already constructed. The purpose of the outline is to help the writer develop the topic.

3. Read Carefully

Following the development of the outline (based on your knowledge of the materials gained in Section A) with a second and more careful reading of the collected materials is a must. Here, you should be armed with a good supply of note cards. At each opportunity, when you identify something of noteworthy importance to the topic at hand, it should be written down. One quotation or one notation per card—never two or more! This is the wisest rule to follow because later the researcher who has recorded two or three important quotations on a single card may find that one quotation will go in one stack for one point and another quotation (from the same card) will need to go in another stack for a different point. One note per card is imperative.

Furthermore, on each card indicate in the top left-hand corner the author, short-word title of the article, and page number. If this information is not written down on each card as the note is being taken, the chances of the card getting mixed up are overwhelming. When the cards are mixed inadvertently, no matter how excellent the information, if the researcher has no idea of the source of the note or the quotation, this particular card is rendered invalid.

4. Revise and Expand

After you have gleaned all the notes and quotations from the materials gathered for the project, the outline developed in Section B must be revised and expanded to incorporate every aspect of the research materials you wish to include. This usually means a minor rewording and/or reworking of the major headings and subheadings, and the further development of subheadings, which will provide a means of incorporating most of the notes and quotations taken in Section C.

5. Cards and Outline

This next to the last step is crucial. Take the outline in its final developed form and place the stack of note cards beside the outline. Holding the stack of cards, label each card in the upper right-hand corner (remember, the author/short title/page number is in the upper left-hand corner) with a Roman numeral corresponding to the major headings of the outline, that is, I, II, III, IV, V, etc. You need to go through the entire stack of cards labeling them with a major heading number and placing each in its appropriate stack.

Now you will have three or four or five large separate stacks of research cards. That task being accomplished, take stack I (the first major division within the outline) and, proceeding through just that stack alone, mark each card with a subheading A, B, C, D, E, etc., which corresponds to the subheadings in the outline under Roman numeral I.

After completing the labeling of the first stack with the subheading letters, proceed to the second and subsequent stacks until all major heading stacks have been divided into the subheading stacks.

Finally, assuming that you have wisely developed subsubheadings, the cards in the subheadings should be divided into subsubheading stacks. (This third level indicates excellence in organization with the subsubheadings often corresponding to individual paragraphs within the finished paper.) That being done, you now have all cards categorized into their appropriate place within the paper. For example, if your paper has three major components I, II, and III, and each of these has three subheadings A, B, C, and each of these has three subsubheadings 1, 2, 3, then you will have divided the research cards first into three stacks corresponding to I, II, III, and then into nine stacks corresponding to I.A, I.B, I.C, II.A, II.B, II.C, III.A, III.B, and III.C. Finally, you will then subdivide these nine stacks into three stacks each corresponding to I.A.1, I.A.2, I.A.3, I.B.1, I.B.2, I.B.3, etc. The smaller the stack, the smaller the category of treatment, thereby making the paper develop in its writing in small careful steps versus wild sporadic steps undisciplined by an outline and organized note cards. (The reason for placing only one bit of information on a single card and identifying that card with author/title/page now has become apparent.)

6. Number the Cards

Now, turn the cards over and number them consecutively from the first to the very last card. Since they are in exactly the proper order for the writing, this precautionary measure is strictly protective. Now, if they are dropped on the floor or mixed up, they can easily and quickly be put back into their proper sequencing.

7. Write the Paper

This, of course, is the whole purpose of the exercise. Line the cards up consecutively, beginning with number one. Put the information from each card, whether note or quotation, into a coherent style of writing, quoting where needed and paraphrasing otherwise. In no time at all the paper is completed and a successful research project brought to completion.

Chapter Seven

A Review of the Process

Like sports, music, art, or any other skill, research and writing are talents that must be developed. The steps outlined here are just the beginning and give only a few of many possible techniques. But by following these recommendations, the researcher can work toward developing the process that best meets his needs.

We have suggested the following steps:

The first step—for those with access to a library—is to become acquainted with the facility well in advance of beginning your research. Get to know its collection, its catalog, its layout, and its staff. This process will save many steps and much valuable time when writing under the pressure of a deadline that often accompanies a research project.

Next, learn how to use the library catalog most effectively and to read and interpret individual catalog records. Each entry in the catalog, whether on paper or online, can be a valuable link to many pieces of information on similar topics. Expert researchers make it a priority to master the library catalog, as they understand that it is a vital information tool.

Learn to use the library's reference collection. Public libraries and academic libraries have different foci, and their reference collections will differ accordingly. While a library specializing in the researcher's subject area will be most valuable, there are resources within any library that can be of great benefit if the researcher will take the time to learn how to properly use the available materials.

Remember that the best and most current research is usually based on the most recent information, which is found in the body of periodical literature, particularly the professional journals. In recent times this body of literature has expanded to include electronic sources as well as print. Both types should be used.

Today's researcher must learn to use the Internet and the many doors it opens, being especially careful to apply good judgment to the validity of sources. While much misinformation and even disinformation appears in print, there is much more of this type of material readily available in the mostly uncontrolled world of the

Internet and the World Wide Web. Used properly, the electronic media can not only lead the researcher to many valuable sources of information but may actually provide the information itself. Combining the use of the Net and the Web with a good document delivery service gives today's researcher more information than has been available to any previous generation—and more quickly.

Always find the best and most appropriate information. Don't be locked into thinking that the best source is always in print or is always electronic. Either type of source can be good or bad, depending upon the information itself and the qualifications of its creator and the needs of the researcher.

Once the information has been gathered, it is the responsibility of the researcher to manage and manipulate that information into a coherent and logical form that supports his thesis. The technique described in Chapter 6 is only one of many. The researcher should take bits and pieces from as many techniques as he has available and mold them into whatever technique works best for him in his own research.

Find the research and writing techniques that work best for you. No one technique will meet the needs of every researcher, nor will a single technique always meet the needs of a given researcher. The more time you spend researching and writing, the better you will become at the process.

In this short book, we have given you only the basics and a few research techniques, but by following these suggestions, you can put together a research project of more-than-acceptable quality. By building on this foundation, you can become a skilled researcher.

Resources

Dictionaries

Bullough, V. L. et al., eds. *American Nursing: A Biographical Dictionary*. New York: Garland, 1988–2000.

Dorland's Illustrated Medical Dictionary. Philadelphia: Saunders, 1900–.

Jablonski, S., ed. *Dictionary of Medical Acronyms and Abbreviations*. 4th ed. Philadelphia: Hanley and Belfus, 2001.

Magalini, S. I., and Magalini, S. C., eds. *Dictionary of Medical Syndromes*. 4th ed. Philadelphia: Lippincott-Raven, 1997.

Melloni, B. J., et al. *Melloni's Illustrated Dictionary of Medical Abbreviations*. New York: Parthenon, 1998.

Melloni, J. L., et al., eds. *Melloni's Illustrated Dictionary of Obstetrics and Gynecology*. New York: Parthenon, 2000.

Miller, Benjamin Frank and Clair Brackman Keane. *Miller-Keane Encyclopedia & Dictionary of Medicine, Nursing, & Allied Health*. 7th ed. Philadelphia: W.B. Saunders, 2003.

Mosby's Medical, Nursing, and Allied Health Dictionary. 6th ed. St. Louis: C.V. Mosby, 2002.

Powers, B. A., and Knapp, T. R. *A Dictionary of Nursing Theory and Research*. 2nd ed. Thousand Oaks, CA: Sage Publications, 1995.

Stanaszek, M. J., et al. *The Inverted Medical Dictionary: A Method of Finding Medical Terms Quickly*. Westport, CT: Technomic, 1991.

Stedman, T. L. *Stedman's Abbreviations, Acronyms, and Symbols*. 3rd ed. Philadelphia: Lippincott Williams & Wilkins, 2003.

Stedman, T. L. *Stedman's Medical Dictionary*. 27th ed. Philadelphia: Lippincott Williams & Wilkins, 2000. *(Also available on CD-ROM.)*

Taber's Cyclopedic Medical Dictionary. Philadelphia: F.A. Davis, 1940–.

Document Delivery Suppliers

Specialized

Business

Technical Information Service, http://www.tis.purdue.edu/TIS

FIND/SVP: Business Research, Consulting and Management Advisory Services, http://www.findsvp.com

HBS Publishing: Harvard Business Review, http://www.hbsp.harvard.edu/products/hbr

Capitol District Information, Inc. (CDI), http://www.capitoldistrict.com

Chemistry

ChemPort, http://www.chemport.org

ChemWeb, http://www.ChemWeb.com

Computing

ACM: Digital Library, http://www.acm.org/dl

Dissertations

ProQuest Digital Dissertations, http://wwwlib.umi.com/dissertations

ProQuest Online Dissertation Services, http://www.umi.com/hp/Products/Dissertations.html

Dissertation Express, http://www.umi.com/hp/Products/DisExpress.html

Legal

Research Associates, http://www.researchassociates.net

Newspapers

NewsLibrary Search, http://www.newslibrary.com

NewsDirectory.com, http://www.newsdirectory.com

Patents

Polyresearch Service—Patent information services and searches, http://www. polyresearch.com

Science

ISI Document Solution: Institute for Scientific Information, http://www.isinet.com/isi/products/ids/ids

Technical Information Service, http://www.ecn.purdue.edu/TIS

HighWire Press, http://highwire.stanford.edu

Buy An Article, http://ojps.aip.org/documentstore/index.jsp

National Agricultural Library Document Delivery Service, http://www.nal.usda.gov/ddsb

Medical

Biomedical Information Service, http://www.biomed.lib.umn.edu/bis

BioMedNet, http://www.bmn.com

foi Online, http://www.foiservices.com

Instant Information Systems, http://www.docdel.com

MedBioWorld, http://www.medbioworld.com

Technology

Technical Information Service, http://www.ecn.purdue.edu/TIS

General

The Digital Vault Initiative, http://www.il.proquest.com/hp/Features/DVault

Teldan Information Systems Ltd., http://www.teldan.co.il/docdeliv.html

TDI Library Services, Inc., http://www.tdico.com

BLPC Ordering, http://blpc.bl.uk

Northern Light, http://www.nlsearch.com

Infotrieve Online, http://www3.infotrieve.com

Information Resource Services, Inc., http://www.librarianoncall.com

Information Prime NA, Inc, http://www.infoprime.com

Infocus Research Services, http://www.infocus-research.com

InfoWorks Technology Company, http://www.itcompany.com

Ingenta, http://www.ingenta.com

New York Public Library Research Libraries, http://www.nypl.org/express

Electric Library Personal Edition, http://www.elibrary.com

ASM International, http://www.asm-intl.org

F.Y.I—County of Los Angeles Public Library, http://www.colapublib.org/fyi.html

The Research Investment, Inc., http://www.researchinvest.com/document_delivery.htm

Doc Deliver, http://www.docdeliver.com

Carolina Library Services, http://www.intrex.net/carolib

Cal Info, http://www.calinfo.net

Cadence Group, http://www.cadence-group.com

Kessler-Hancock, http://www.khinfo.com

The British Library, http://www.bl.uk

Advanced Information Consultants, http://www.advinfoc.com

U. of Washington Libraries Research Express, http://www.lib.washington.edu/Resxp

Instant Information Systems, http://www.docdel.com

Outside the U.S

HighWire Press, http://www.highwire.org

Asia
Japan
Infonetwork, http://www.doc-quest.com

Australia
express Information, http://www.expressinfo.com.au/research.html

National Library of Australia Document Supply Service, http://www.nla.gov.au/dss

MONINFO Home (Monash University), http://www.lib.monash.edu.au/moninfo

Rapid Services—UNSW, http://www.library.unsw.edu.au/rapid.html

Europe

Austria

Central Library for Physics in Vienna, http://www.univie.ac.at/zbph

Zentralbibliothek für Physik in Wien, http://www.zbp.univie.ac.at/edefault.htm

England

IEE Library Services, http://www.iee.org/TheIEE/Research/LibSvc

British Library Document Supply Centre, http://www.bl.uk/services/bsds/dsc/delivery.html

Finland

Helsinki School of Economics Library, http://helecon.hkkk.fi/library

Germany

DBI-LINK die Verbindung zwischen Benutzer und Bibliothek, http://www.dbilink.de/en

German National Library of Medicine—Cologne, http://www.zbmed.de/english/dv_allg_eng.html

The Broker Research Center—Delivery of patent copies, http://www.infobroker.de/service/patdele.html

Ireland

University of Limerick's Business & Technical Information Service (BTIS), http://www.btis.ie

Italy

Quaestio- Information Broker, http://www.quaestio.it

Netherlands

AGRALIN home page, http://www.bib.wau.nl

Polyresearch Service—Patent information services and searches, http://www.polyresearch.com

The NIWI Web Site, http://www.niwi.knaw.nl

Inhoud van de NIWI Web Site, http://www.niwi.knaw.nl/nl/homepag.htm

NIWI Web Site [English], http://www.niwi.knaw.nl/us/homepag.htm

Russia

Access Russia Information Services, http://www.arussia.com

Russian Periodicals Online, http://www.russianstory.com

Scotland

Recal Information Services, http://www.recal.org.uk

Latin America

Argentina

Ontyme Information Brokers, http://www.informar.com.ar

Middle East

Israel

Infomayda, http://www.actcom.co.il/~atoz

North America

Canada

Canada Institute for Scientific and Technical Information (CISTI), http://www.nrc.ca/cisti/docdel/docdel_e.shtml

Micromedia ProQuest, http://www.micromedia.on.ca

Encyclopedias

Encyclopedia of Nursing Research. Joyce J. Fitzpatrick, ed. New York: Springer, 1998.

Gale Encyclopedia of Nursing & Allied Health. Detroit: Gale Group, 2002.

Mezey, Mathy Doval. *The Encyclopedia of Elder Care: the comprehensive resource on geriatric and social care.* New York: Springer, 2001.

Nurse's Book of Advice: An Encyclopedia of Answers to Hundreds of Difficult Questions-Ethical, Legal, Moral, Technical, and Professional. Springhouse, PA: Springhouse, 1992.

Schroeder, Patricia. *Encyclopedia of Nursing Care Quality.* Boston: Jones & Bartlett, 1995.

Who's Who in American Nursing. New Providence, NJ: Marquis, 1984–.

Lexicons, Yearbooks, and Handbooks

AACN's Clinical Reference for Critical Care Nursing. 4th ed., edited by Marguerite Rodgers Kinney et al. St. Louis: Mosby, 1998.

Annual Review of Nursing Research. New York: Springer, 1983–.

Carpenito, Lynda Juall. *Handbook of Nursing Diagnosis.* 9th ed. Philadelphia: Lippincott, 2002.

Clinical Nursing Skills and Techniques. 5th ed. Anne G. Perry and Patricia A. Potter, eds. St. Louis: Mosby, 2002. [Available on CD-ROM]

Dudek, Susan G. *Nutrition Essential for Nursing Practice.* 4th ed. Philadelphia: Lippincott, 2001.

Dufour, D. Robert. *Clinical Use of Laboratory Data: A Practical Guide.* Baltimore: Williams & Wilkins, 1998.

Facts About Nursing. New York: American Nurses' Association, 1935–.

Handbook of Clinical Nursing Research. Thousand Oaks, CA: Sage, 1999.

The Lippincott Manual of Nursing Practice. Philadelphia: Lippincott, 2001.

The Merck Manual of Medical Information. Whitehouse Station, NJ: Merck Research Laboratories, 2003.

Nursing Diagnosis Handbook: A guide to planning care. Ackley, B. J., et al. 5th ed. St. Louis: Mosby, 2002.

Sacher, Ronald A., et al. *Widmann's Clinical Interpretation of Laboratory Tests.* 11th ed. Philadelphia: Davis, 2000.

Other References

Andriot, J. L., et al. *Guide to U. S. Government Publications*. Farmington Hills, MI: Gale Group, 1973–.

Brink, Pamela J. *Basic Steps in Planning Nursing Research: From Question to Proposal*. 5th ed. Boston: Jones and Bartlett, 2001.

Bullough, Bonnie. *Nursing, a Historical Bibliography*. New York: Garland, 1981.

Burkhardt, Margaret A. and Alvita K. Nathaniel. *Ethics & Issues in Contemporary Nursing*. 2nd ed. Australia; Albany: Delmar/Thomson Learning, 2002.

Burns, Nancy. *The Practice of Nursing Research: Conduct, Critique, & Utilization*. 4th ed. Philadelphia: Saunders, 2001.

Clamp, Cynthia G. L. and Stephen Gough. *Resources for Nursing Research: An Annotated Bibliography*. 3rd ed. Thousand Oaks, CA: Sage, 1999.

Dempsey, Patricia Ann and Arthur D. Dempsey. *Using Nursing Research: Process, Critical Evaluation, and Utilization*. Baltimore, MD: Jones and Bartlett, 2000.

Fitzpatrick, Joyce J. and Kristen S. Montgomery. *Maternal Child Health Nursing Research Digest*. New York: Springer, 1999.

Gates, Jean Key. *Guide to the Use of Libraries and Information Sources*. 7th ed. New York: McGraw-Hill, 1994.

Hott, Jacqueline Rose, Wendy C. Budin, and Lucille E. Notter. *Notter's Essentials of Nursing Research*. 6th ed. New York: Springer, 1999.

Instruments for Clinical Health-care Research. 2nd ed. Boston: Jones and Bartlett, 1997. *(Also available in electronic format.)*

Morehead, Joe. *Introduction to United States Public Documents*. 3rd ed. Littleton, CO: Libraries Unlimited, Inc., 1983.

Munhall, Patricia L. *Qualitative Research Proposals and Reports: A Guide*. 2nd ed. Sudbury, MA: Jones and Bartlett, 2000.

Nieswiadomy, Rose Marie. *Foundations of Nursing Research*. 4th ed. Upper Saddle River, NJ: Prentice Hall, 2002.

Nursing Research: A Qualitative Perspective. 3rd ed. Sudbury, MA: Jones and Bartlett, 2001.

Nursing Research: Methods, Critical Appraisal, and Utilization, 5th ed. St. Louis: Mosby, 2001.

Polit, Denise F., Cheryl Tatano Beck, and Bernadette P. Hungler. *Essentials of Nursing Research: Methods and Applications*. 5th ed. Philadelphia: Lippincott, 2001.

The Research Process in Nursing. Desmond F. S. Cormak, ed. Oxford: Blackwell Science, 2000.

Rice, Virginia Hill. *Handbook of Stress, Coping, and Health.* Thousand Oaks, CA: Sage, 2000.

Ross, Linda A. *Nurses' Perceptions of Spiritual Care.* Brookfield, VT: Avebury, 1997.

Schmeckebier, Laurence F. and Roy B. Eastin. *Government Publications and Their Use.* 2nd rev. ed. Washington: The Brookings Institution, 1986.

Young, Anne, Susan Gebhardt Taylor, and Katherine McLaughlin-Renpenning. *Connections: Nursing Research, Theory, and Practice.* St. Louis: Mosby, 2001.

Indexes

Bibliographic Index. [New York]: H.W. Wilson Co., 1938–.

Biography Index. New York: H.W. Wilson Co., 1946–.

Book Review Digest. New York: H.W. Wilson Company, 1905–.

Book Review Index. Detroit: Gale Research Co., 1965–.

Cumulative Index to Nursing Literature. Glendale, CA: Seventh Day Adventist Hospital Association, 1961–1976.

Cumulative Index to Nursing and Allied Health Literature. Glendale, CA: Glendale Adventist Medical Center, 1977–.

Current Book Review Citations. New York: H.W. Wilson Co., 1976–1982.

Humanities Index. New York: H.W. Wilson Co., 1974–.

Index to U. S. Government Periodicals. [Chicago]: Infordata International, 1970–1987.

International Nursing Index. New York: American Journal of Nursing, 1966–.

Nursing Studies Index. Yale University, School of Nursing. Philadelphia: Lippincott, 1963–1972.

PAIS International (Public Affairs Information Service Bulletin). New York: Public Affairs Information Service, 1991–.

Readers' Guide to Periodical Literature. New York: H.W. Wilson Co., 1901–.

Social Sciences Index. New York: H.W. Wilson Co., 1974–.

Major Nursing and Health Sciences Periodicals

AACN Clinical Issues

AORN Journal—Association of Operating Room Nurses Journal

Advances in Nursing Science

Canadian Journal of Psychiatric Nursing

Canadian Nurse

Cancer Nursing: An International Journal for Cancer Research

Cardiovascular Nursing

Critical Care Nursing Quarterly

DCCN: Dimension of Critical Care Nursing

Home Healthcare Nurse

Image: The Journal of Nursing Scholarship

Imprint (National Student Nurses Association)

International Nursing Review

Issues in Comprehensive Pediatric Nursing

Issues in Mental Health Nursing

Journal of Advanced Nursing

Journal of Christian Nursing

Journal of Continuing Education in Nursing

Journal of Gerontological Nursing

Journal of Neuroscience Nursing

Journal of Nursing Administration

Journal of Nursing Education

Journal of Psychosocial Nursing and Mental Health Services

MCN: The American Journal of Maternal Child Nursing

Maternal-Child Nursing Journal

Nurse Practitioner

Nurse, Patient and the Law

Nursing Administration Quarterly

Nursing Clinics of North America

Nursing Economics

Nursing Management

Nursing Times

Oncology Nursing Forum

Orthopaedic Nursing

Pediatric Nursing

Research in Nursing and Health

Topics in Clinical Nursing

Western Journal of Nursing Research

Stylesheets for Citing Electronic Information

American Medical Association. *American Medical Association Manual of Style: Guide for Authors and Editors.* 9th ed. Baltimore: Williams & Wilkins, 1998.

American Psychological Association. *Publication Manual of the American Psychological Association.* 5th ed. Washington, DC: The Association, 2001.

Barnum, B. *Writing and Getting Published: A Primer for Nurses.* New York: Springer, 1995.

Bradigan, P. S., et al. *Writer's Guide to Nursing and Allied Health Journals.* Washington, DC: American Nurses Publishing, 1998.

Chicago Manual of Style: The Essential Guide for Authors, Editors and Publishers. 15th ed. Chicago: University of Chicago Press, 2003.

Fondiller, S. H. *The Writer's Workbook: Health Professionals Guide to Getting Published.* 2nd ed. Sudbury, MA: Jones and Bartlett, 1999. *(Also available in electronic format).*

Gibaldi, Joseph. *MLA Handbook for Writers of Research Papers.* 6th ed., New York: Modern Language Association of America, 2003.

Greenhill, Anita. *Electronic References & Scholarly Citations of Internet Sources.* Queensland: Griffith University, 1995. *(Also available in electronic format.)*

Harnack, Andrew. *Beyond the MLA Handbook: Documenting Electronic Sources on the Internet*. Richmond, KY: Eastern Kentucky University, 1999. *(Also available in electronic format.)*

Huth, E. J. *Writing and Publishing in Medicine*. 3rd ed. Baltimore: Williams & Wilkins, 1999.

Li, Xia, and Nancy Crane. *Electronic Styles: A Handbook for Citing Electronic Information*. 2nd ed. Medford, NJ: Information Today, 1996.

Sheridan D. R, and Dowdney, D. L. *How to Write and Publish Articles in Nursing*. 2nd ed. New York: Springer, 1997.

Thibault, Danielle. *Bibliographic Style Manual*. Ottawa: National Library of Canada, 1998.

Turabian, K. L. *A Manual for Writers of Term Papers, Theses, and Dissertations*. 6th ed. Chicago: University of Chicago Press, 1996.

Walker, Janice R. *The Columbia Guide to Online Style*. New York: Columbia University Press, 1998.

Walker, Janice R. *MLA-Style Citations of Electronic Sources*. Tampa, FL: Janice R. Walker, 1995. *(Also available in electronic format.)*

Winkler, Anthony C. *Writing the Research Paper: A Handbook with Both the MLA and APA Documentation Styles*. 5th ed. Fort Worth: Harcourt Brace College Publishers, 1999.

Internet and Online Resources

Books and Bookstores

Amazon.com, http://www.amazon.com

Barnes and Noble, http://www.barnesandnoble.com

Bartleby.com Great Books Online, http://www.bartleby.com

Bibliofind, http://www.bibliofind.com

Blackwell's, http://bookshop.blackwells.co.uk

The Bookpl@ce, http://www.thebookplace.com

Bookwire, http://www.bookwire.com

Borders, http://www.borders.com

Internet bookshop, http://www.bookshop.co.uk

Project Gutenberg, http://promo.net/pg

Waterstone's, http://www.waterstones.co.uk

Community Networks

Michiana Free-Net, http://michiana.org

Chicago Mosaic, http://www.ci.chi.il.us

San Diego Source, http://www.sddt.com

Austin Free-Net, http://www.austinfree.net

Databases

The Internet Movie Database, http://www.imdb.com

Gracenote, http://www.gracenote.com

Dictionaries

The LOGOS Dictionary, http://www.logos.it

OneLook Dictionaries, http://www.onelook.com

Merriam-Webster, http://www.m-w.com

Roget's Thesaurus, http://thesaurus.com

The Semantic Rhyming Dictionary, http://www.rhymezone.com

A Web of On-line Dictionaries, http://www.yourdictionary.com

Government Resources

Federal Citizen Information Center (FIC), http://fic.info.gov

FedWorld, http://www.fedworld.gov

United States Government Printing Office, http://www.gpoaccess.gov

U. S. Census Bureau, http://www.census.gov

U. S. Senate, http://www.senate.gov

U. S. House, http://www.house.gov

The White House, http://www.whitehouse.gov

CCTA Information Service, http://www.open.gov.uk

Libraries and Library Networks

Library of Congress, http://www.loc.gov

The British Library, http://portico.bl.uk

National Library of Canada, http://www.nlc-bnc.ca

SAILOR, Maryland's Public Information Network, http://www.sailor.lib.md.us

ACLIN, Access Colorado Library and Information Network, http://www.aclin.org

Galileo, Georgia's Virtual Library, http://www.galileo.usg.edu

INSPIRE, Indiana Virtual Library, http://www.inspire.net

Internet Public Library, http://www.ipl.org

Miscellaneous

Bartlett's Familiar Quotations, http://www.bartleby.com/100

Harvard Business School, http://www.hbs.harvard.edu

Newsgroups and Mailing Lists

Google Groups, http://groups.google.com

Liszt (Now Topica), http://www.liszt.com

Organizations

American Cancer Society, http://www.cancer.org

American Heart Association, http://www.americanheart.org

American Medical Association, http://www.ama-assn.org

American Psychological Association, http://www.apa.org

Radio and TV Stations

Broadcast.com, http://broadcast.com

Nursing Resources

Allnurses.com, http://allnurses.com

American Association for Colleges of Nursing, http://www.aacn.nche.edu

American Nursing Association's Nursing World, http://www.nursingworld.org

Canadian Nurses' Association, http://www.cna-nurses.ca

Canadian Nursing Index, http://nursingindex.com

CliniWeb International, http://www.ohsu.edu/cliniweb

DelmarHealthCare.com, http://www.delmarhealthcare.com

Hardin Meta Directory of Health Internet Sites, http://www.lib.uiowa.edu/hardin/md

HealthWeb, http://healthweb.org

Interagency Council on Information Resources for Nursing, http://www.icirn.org

NursingCenter, http://www.nursingcenter.com

National Institute of Nursing Research, http://www.nih.gov/ninr

National League for Nursing, http://www.nln.org

National Library of Medicine, http://www.nlm.nih.gov

NMAP, http://nmap.ac.uk

NP Central, http://www.npcentral.net

Nurse.org, http://www.nurse.org

NursingNet, http://www.nursingnet.org

Nursing Network, http://www.nursingnetwork.com

Nursing Network Humor Page, http://www.nursingnetwork.com/humor.htm

Nursing Standard, http://www.nursing-standard.co.uk

Nursing Theory Page, http://www.sandiego.edu/nursing/theory

Nursing Websearch, http://www.nursingwebsearch.com

Nursing World, http://nursingworld.org

Online Journal of Issues in Nursing, http://nursingworld.org/ojin

RN Central, http://www.rncentral.com

Sigma Theta Tau International, http://www.nursingsociety.org

U. of Buffalo Selected Nursing Web Sites, http://ublib.buffalo.edu/libraries/units/hsl/internet/nsgsites.html

Virtual Nurse, http://virtualnurse.com

Search Engines (General)

About.com, http://www.about.com

Altavista, http://www.altavista.com

Excite, http://www.excite.com

Go.com, http://infoseek.go.com

Google, http://www.google.com

HotBot, http://hotbot.lycos.com

LookSmart, http://www.looksmart.com

Lycos, http://www.Lycos.com

Netscape Search, http://search.netscape.com

Northern Light, http://www.nlsearch.com

Overture, http://www.overture.com

Teoma, http://www.teoma.com

Thunderstone, http://www.thunderstone.com

Webcrawler, http://www.webcrawler.com

Yahoo!, http://www.yahoo.com

Search Engines (Specialized)

DevX, http://www.devx.com

EarthCam, http://www.earthcam.com

Google Groups, http://groups.google.com

Search Engines (Metasearch)

Dogpile, http://www.dogpile.com

Metacrawler, http://www.metacrawler.com

Webrings

WebRing, http://www.webring.com

The Rail, http://www.therail.com

Bomis.com, http://www.bomis.com

About the Authors

Dennis C. Tucker has worked in libraries of many types and sizes, including the Mishawka (Indiana) Public Library and the University of Notre Dame. He served for over a decade at Indiana Cooperative Library Services Authority (INCOLSA) in a variety of positions. He holds an M.A.T. from Southeast Missouri State University, an M.L.S. from the University of Missouri, and a Ph.D. from Foundation House/Oxford. Tucker and Craig were collaborators at Northwestern State University of Louisiana, where she was Head of the Library at the School of Nursing and he, Director of Libraries. Tucker is the author of several well-reviewed books including *Research Techniques for Scholars and Students in Religion and Theology* and *Library Relocations and Collection Shifts*.

Paula Craig is E-Learning Coordinator for Weill Cornell Medical College in Doha, Qatar. With more than 33 years of experience in health science libraries, including her time as the Head of the Library at Northwestern State University College of Nursing, Craig has developed and taught many medical and health online literature classes. She was director of the Library at Christus Schumpert Medical Center and coordinator of Continuing Medical Education at Louisiana State University Health Science Center in Shreveport, Louisiana. For many years Craig served as Associate Director of MD Anderson Cancer Center Library. She has also been a consultant for health related-issues to the legal profession for many years. She holds a Masters degree in Library and Information Science from the University of Oklahoma in Norman, Oklahoma.

Index

A

B

C

More Titles of Interest

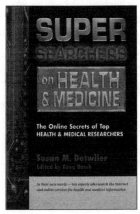

Super Searchers on Health and Medicine

Susan M. Detwiler; edited by Reva Basch

With human lives depending on them, skilled medical researchers rank among the best online searchers in the world. In *Super Searchers on Health & Medicine*, medical librarians, clinical researchers, health information specialists, and physicians explain how they combine traditional sources with the best of the Net to deliver just what the doctor ordered. If you use the Internet and online databases to answer important health and medical questions, these super searchers will help guide you around the perils and pitfalls to the best sites, sources, and techniques.

Softbound • ISBN 0-910965-44-7
$24.95

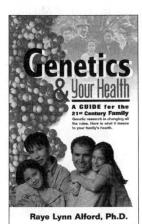

Genetics and Your Health

Raye Lynn Alford, Ph.D.

Public interest in genetics has never been greater now that gene research promises to revolutionize medicine in the 21st century. In addition to the medical applications, the confidentiality of information and regulation of genetic technologies are hot-button topics. *Genetics and Your Health* will answer your questions about what the startling advances in genetic research, testing, and therapy really mean to today's family. Included is a directory to medical resources for genetics care, support, and information over the internet, and a chapter devoted to the Human Genome Project.

Hardbound • ISBN 0-9666748-2-0 • $29.95
Softbound • ISBN 0-9666748-1-2 • $19.95

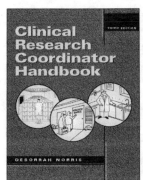

Clinical Research Coordinator Handbook, 3rd Ed.

Deborrah Norris

In this revised third edition of the essential reference for clinical research coordinators (CRCs), Deborrah Norris provides expanded coverage of CRC duties and regulatory requirements, including new sections on investigator responsibilities, data clarification, and adverse event reporting. The book's five appendices include a directory of CRC resources, updated forms and checklists, state regulatory requirements and contact information, conversion charts and tables, a glossary, and more.

Softbound • ISBN 0-937548-54-5
$39.95

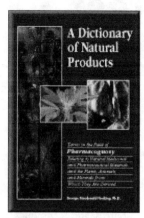

A Dictionary of Natural Products

George Macdonald Hocking, Ph.D.

A Dictionary of Natural Products is primarily devoted to an arrangement and explanation of terms relating to natural, non-artificial crude drugs from the vegetable, animal, and mineral kingdoms. This volume presents over 18,000 entries of medicinal, pharmaceutical, and related products appearing on the market as raw materials or occurring in drug stores, folk medical practice, and in chemical manufacturing processes.

Hardbound • ISBN 0-937548-31-6
$139.50

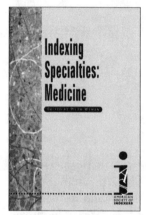

Indexing Speciaties: Medicine

Edited by Pilar Wyman

This in-depth look at the indexing specialty field of medicine includes contributions from more than a dozen noted medical indexers. The book features 13 chapters and four parts: "Medical Indexers," "Medical Indexes," "Medical Indexing," and "Resources." A directory of medical reference tools and Internet sites is included.

Softbound • ISBN 1-57387-02-X
$35.00

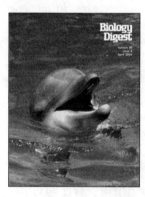

Biology Digest

Biology Digest is a comprehensive abstracts journal covering all the life sciences. Each monthly issue contains more than 300 abstracts which are, in essence, individual digests of articles and research reports gathered from worldwide sources. Important information is retained in the abstracts to give a precise, inclusive summary of the original material.

Biology Digest was specially created to meet the needs of high school and undergraduate college students and is now used in more than 3,000 schools worldwide. It provides easy access to new scientific developments at a comprehension level appropriate for students. However, *Biology Digest* has proved to be useful to biologists at all levels—professional and amateur alike.

Biology Digest and its companion databases are available electronically through a special arrangement with NewsBank, Inc. For more information on the ScienceSource Collection, contact NewsBank, Inc. at (800) 762-8182, or e-mail sales@newsbank.com.

ISSN 0095-2958 • 1 year $149.00